Aids to Postgraduate Medicine

Aids to Postgraduate Medicine

J. L. Burton

M.D., B.Sc., F.R.C.P.
Consultant Senior Lecturer in Dermatology
Bristol Royal Infirmary

Third Edition

CHURCHILL LIVINGSTONE
EDINBURGH LONDON AND NEW YORK 1978

CHURCHILL LIVINGSTONE
Medical Division of Longman Group Limited

Distributed in the United States of America by
Longman Inc., 19 West 44th Street, New York,
N.Y. 10036 and by associated companies,
branches and representatives throughout the
world.

First Edition   1970
  Reprinted   1970
  Reprinted   1971
  Reprinted   1972
Second Edition   1974
  Reprinted   1976
Third Edition   1978

ISBN 0 443 01812 X

British Library Cataloguing in Publication Data
Burton, John Lloyd
  Aids to postgraduate medicine. – 3rd ed
  1. Pathology   2. Medicine
  I. Title
  616   RB111   78–40029

Printed in Singapore by
Kyodo-Shing Loong Printing Industries Pte Ltd

Preface to third edition

This book is intended primarily to provide a compact aid to revision for candidates taking postgraduate examinations such as the M.R.C.P. (U.K.). I hope it will also prove useful to other doctors wishing quickly to refresh their memory of the diagnostic possibilities in a particular case.

This edition has been completely revised, and a considerable amount of new material has been added. Some of the lists have been derived from the textbooks named in the Bibliography, but the majority have come from the excellent review articles which now appear regularly in the journals and annual books devoted to postgraduate education. Many of the lists are followed by suggestions for further reading, so that this book should serve as a readily available source of reference to articles which will provide a comprehensive review as well as an introduction to the original literature.

I should like to thank the many people who have suggested improvements to this book, and I am particularly indebted to many of my consultant colleagues in the Bristol Health District who have given me much helpful advice and constructive criticism.

Keeping this book up-to-date is like taking the M.R.C.P. examination at three yearly intervals, and so I should also like to acknowledge the encouragement I have received from the many examination candidates who have been kind enough to say they have found the book useful. It is too much to hope that this new edition will make enjoyable reading, but I hope that future readers will at least find it equally helpful.

1978   J.L.B.

Contents

The M.R.C.P. examination   1
Cardiology   3
Chest disease   20
Gastroenterology   37
Haematology   63
Neurology   92
Endocrine and bone disease   118
Renal disease   138
Rheumatology   153
Dermatology   167
Immunology   183
Genetics   188
Microbiology   192
Clinical chemistry   194
Bibliography   198
Index   201
Notes

The M.R.C.P. examination

The Royal College of Physicians held a Symposium in 1977 to explain some recent changes in the M.R.C.P. examination. The published proceedings (*Brit. Med. J.* (1978) **1**, 217) may be summarized as follows:

The Part I examination. This is designed to filter off candidates who are insufficiently prepared for the Part II examination. Only about one-third of candidates pass the Part I examination each year.

Candidates are advised to prepare by wide reading of textbooks and monographs, particularly on the main themes relevant to clinical practice in Britain. Questions are asked about common and important topics, and also about areas of new knowledge.

Each paper has 60 questions, selected from a bank of about 4000 questions and over 100 new questions are added to the bank each year. The distribution of the 60 questions is as follows:

Cardiology	4	Clinical pharmacology	5
Respiratory	4	Symptoms and signs	1 or 2
Gastroenterology	4	Endocrinology	3
Tropical	1 or 0	Renal disease	3
Statistics	1	Muscular and skeletal	2
Anatomy	1	Reticuloendothelial	1
Physiology	1	Toxicology	1
Neurology	4	Immunology and allergy	1 or 2
Haematology	2 or 3	Industrial medicine	1
Dermatology	1	Metabolic disease	2
Venereology	1	Genetics	1
Paediatrics	4	Ophthalmology	1
Psychiatry	4	Infectious disease	2 or 3

The multiple true-false format is used, with five items in each question. The marking is +1 for a correct answer, –1 for a wrong answer, and 0 for 'don't know'. Candidates often look for subtlety that is not intended by the examiner and each question should be taken at its face value. Variation in standards from year to year is checked by using in each paper 6 to 10 marker questions which have been used before.

The Part II examination. Like Part I, this is a test of knowledge, but in addition it tests skill in history-taking and physical examination, judgement and attitudes (e.g. is the candidate kind and considerate?).

Essay questions are no longer used, because their marking is subjective and therefore unreliable. The present written paper can be objectively marked. Each question has an accepted answer, but the examiners are allowed to use their own judgement in giving appropriate marks if the candidate has given some other answer. Candidates have to answer questions on diagnosis and investigation following 4 case-histories (with no choice), and 10 data interpretations. The latter include electrocardiograms, but are mainly laboratory data. There are also questions on 20 projected slides (or pairs of slides). Each is shown for 90 seconds, after which a bell rings, and another 30 seconds is then allowed before the slide is changed. When slides of the fundi are shown, a picture of a normal fundus is first projected and photographic artefacts are pointed out.

The long case tests skill in history-taking and physical examination. The examiners recognize that the long case, especially the history, is probably the least valid part of the examination because so much depends on the individual patient. The short cases (usually only 3) probably give the examiners a better idea of the candidate's skill in physical examination. The candidate is examined by two examiners for 20 minutes on each occasion.

The oral examination is not simply a test of knowledge, but is supposed to find out how a candidate reacts to certain clinical situations and whether he understands basic principles. The oral examination has 2 examiners plus the possibility of a third specialist examiner. Two examiners each examine the candidate for 10 minutes.

Marks are allocated in the Part II examination in the proportion of two for the written paper, two for the clinical and one for the oral, but no candidate can pass if he fails the clinical examination.

Candidates can now take the whole of Part II either in general medicine or in paediatrics.

Cardiology

AUSCULTATION
HEART SOUNDS

1. Valve closure
1st heart sound (mitral and tricuspid valves)
  (i) Loud in: Mitral stenosis
                Hyperdynamic circulation
                Tachycardia
  (ii) Normally split in tricuspid area on inspiration

2nd heart sound (aortic and pulmonary valves)
  (i) Normally split on inspiration, especially in children
  (ii) Loud narrowly split P_2 in pulmonary hypertension
  (iii) Soft widely split P_2 in pulmonary stenosis
  (iv) Widely split in RBBB
  (v) Widely split fixed P_2 in ASD
  (vi) Paradoxically split P_2 (narrows on inspiration) in LBBB and
       rarely in aortic stenosis and severe hypertension

2. Opening snap
Heard only with AV valve stenosis
Indicates mobile AV valve
Mitral opening snap in mitral stenosis is maximal medial to apex,
louder during expiration, thereby differentiated from split P_2
Closeness to 2nd sound indicates severity of stenosis

3. Ejection sounds
Early systolic clicks due to aortic or pulmonary stenosis, or to
dilatation of pulmonary artery or aorta in pulmonary or systemic
hypertension

4. Ventricular filling sounds (Triple rhythm)

Diastolic sounds are due to:
  (i) 3rd heart sound (rapid ventricular filling)
  (ii) atrial (4th) sound (forceful atrial contraction)
  (iii) summation of both

3rd heart sound is normal in young people. Occurs in older people in:

    (i) R or L ventricular failure
    (ii) Mitral or tricuspid regurgitation
    (iii) Constrictive pericarditis (early and sharp)

Atrial sound is abnormal, occurs in resistance to LV filling e.g. hypertensive LVH, aortic stenosis
Summation sound is normal during tachycardia

5. Extracardiac sounds
Usually pericardial in origin, vary with respiration and posture

HEART MURMURS

High-pitched indicate large pressure difference across small orifice, e.g. AI
Low-pitched indicate small pressure difference across large orifice, e.g. MS

1. Systolic
    (i) Midsystolic ejection murmurs
       Aortic
       a. Aortic stenosis—confirmed by narrow pulse pressure and thrill (patient leaning forward in expiration)
       b. Increased flow rate
       c. Valve thickening or sclerosis without stenosis
       d. Post-valvar dilatation, e.g. hypertension
       Pulmonary
       a. Functional, especially in young people
       b. Pulmonary stenosis
       c. Increased flow rate ASD, TAPVD (total anomalous pulmonary venous drainage), hyperdynamic circulation
       d. Post-valvar dilatation, e.g. pulmonary hypertension or aortic aneurysm
    (ii) Pansystolic murmurs
       Extend from 1st to 2nd sound
       a. Mitral regurgitation—propagated into axilla
       b. Tricuspid regurgitation—increases with inspiration, soft unless pulmonary hypertension is present
       c. VSD—3rd or 4th LICS. Thrill in 90 per cent

Causes of a loud systolic murmur with a thrill
    (i) At apex—mitral regurgitation
    (ii) At 4th LICS—VSD
    (iii) At pulmonary area—pulmonary stenosis
    (iv) At aortic area—aortic stenosis

2. Diastolic
    (i) *Mitral or tricuspid stenosis*
       Degree of stenosis indicated by duration of murmur, not intensity
       Mitral stenosis—use bell, lightly applied at apex, with patient on L side in expiration. Presystolic accentuation is often a sign of pure stenosis, but is absent in atrial fibrillation
       Tricuspid stenosis—murmur louder on inspiration
    (ii) *Mitral or tricuspid thickening* e.g. Carey-Coombs murmur of active rheumatic carditis
    (iii) *Increased AV flow rate*
       Mitral in VSD and PDA (patent ductus arteriosus)
       Tricuspid in ASD and TAPVD
    (iv) *Aortic or pulmonary regurgitation*
       Aortic regurgitation—often missed. Listen with diaphragm all down L sternal edge for soft 'whispered R' murmur with patient leaning forward in expiration
       Pulmonary regurgitation—usually due to pulmonary hypertension
       Austin-Flint murmur (functional mitral stenosis) may occur in Aortic Incompetence
       GrahaM-Steell murmur (pulmonary regurgitation) may occur in Mitral Stenosis with pulmonary hypertension

3. Continuous ('Machinery murmur')
    (i) Patent ductus arteriosus (2nd LICS or under clavicle)
    (ii) Aortico-pulmonary septal defect (2nd or 3rd LICS)
    (iii) Pulmonary AV fistula (over lung fields)
    (iv) Bronchial artery anastomosis in pulmonary atresia
    (v) Artificial ductus (Blalock or Waterston shunt)
    (vi) Venous hum

Effect of respiration on murmurs

Inspiration increases stroke volume of R ventricle, therefore increases intensity of TS, TI and PS

Inspiration increases vascular volume of lungs and decreases stroke volume of L ventricle, therefore decreases intensity of MS, MI, AS and AI

Effect of posture on murmurs and cardiac sounds

Mitral systolic and diastolic murmurs. Accentuated in L lateral position

Aortic murmurs, ejection clicks and pericardial rub. Accentuated when sitting up

Functional systolic murmurs. Accentuated when lying down

Venous hum. Heard only when upright

Effect of drugs on murmurs

Drugs increasing arteriolar resistance will decrease systolic ejection murmurs and increase regurgitant murmurs at all valves

Vasodilators have the opposite effect

Characteristics of innocent systolic murmurs in childhood

1. No other abnormality detected
2. No thrill
3. Usually short, of low frequency, and in early or mid-systole
4. Not localised to a specific area, and not radiating outside praecordium
5. Intensity often varies with change in posture

Further reading

Hamer, J. (1975) *Medicine,* 2nd series, **25,** 1208.
Leatham, A. (1976) *Auscultation of the Heart and Phonocardiography,* 2nd Edn., Edinburgh: Churchill Livingstone.

CAUSES OF VALVULAR DISEASE

1. Congenital
2. Rheumatic
3. Syphilis
4. Infective endocarditis (bacterial or mycotic)
5. Libman-Sach's endocarditis (SLE)
6. Carcinoid
7. Ankylosing spondylitis
8. Marfan's
9. Atheroma
10. Dissecting aneurysm
11. Trauma

Differential diagnosis
1. Functional murmur
2. Atrial myxoma
3. Hypertrophic obstructive cardiomyopathy (HOCM)
4. Ruptured papillary muscle or chordae tendineae
5. Aneurysm of sinus of Valsalva

HEART FAILURE

VALSALVA MANOEUVRE

Normal response of pulse and BP

Cardiac failure causes a square wave response

CAUSES OF LV FAILURE

1. **Pressure overload**
     (i) Hypertension
     (ii) Aortic stenosis
     (iii) Coarctation

2. **Volume overload**
     (i) Aortic or mitral regurgitation
     (ii) VSD or PDA
     (iii) AV fistula or anaemia

3. **Myocardial ischaemia**
     (i) Coronary artery disease
     (ii) Severe anaemia
     (iii) Tachycardia

4. **Primary myocardial disease**
     (i) Myocarditis
     (ii) Cardiomyopathy

CAUSES OF RV FAILURE

1. **Pressure overload**
     (i) Pulmonary hypertension secondary to LVF or MS.
     (ii) Cor pulmonale
     (iii) Severe pulmonary stenosis

2. **Volume overload**
     (i) Tricuspid regurgitation
     (ii) ASD or TAPVD

Further reading
Hamer, J. (1975) *Medicine,* 2nd series, **25**, 1208.

JUGULAR VENOUS PULSE
Normal jugular venous pulse wave

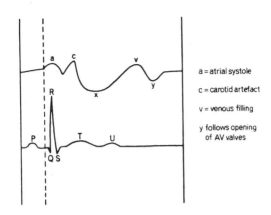

a = atrial systole

c = carotid artefact

v = venous filling

y follows opening
  of AV valves

Abnormalities of venous pulse wave
1. *Giant 'a' waves*
   - (i) pulmonary hypertension
   - (ii) severe pulmonary stenosis
   - (iii) tricuspid stenosis
2. *Cannon waves*
   - (i) Regular: Nodal rhythm
   - (ii) Irregular: Complete heart block
           Multiple extrasystoles
3. *Absent 'a' waves:* atrial fibrillation
4. *Independent 'a' waves:* complete heart block
5. *Large 'v' waves:* tricuspid incompetence (confirm by palpation of systolic impulse in liver)
6. *Deep 'y' descent:* any cause of very high JVP especially constrictive pericarditis
7. *Slow 'y' descent:* tricuspid stenosis

ARTERIAL PULSE

Causes of tachycardia
1. Sinus tachycardia (q.v.)
2. Supraventricular (atrial or nodal) tachycardia
3. Atrial flutter
4. Atrial fibrillation
5. Ventricular tachycardia
6. Ventricular flutter

Causes of sinus tachycardia
1. Hyperdynamic circulation (p. 16)
2. Congestive cardiac failure
3. Constrictive pericarditis
4. Drugs (adrenaline, atropine, nitrites, etc.)
5. Hypovolaemic shock (acute haemorrhage, etc.)

Further reading

Besterman, E. (1975) *Medicine,* 2nd series, **25,** 1200.

Causes of a slow regular pulse
1. Sinus bradycardia (q.v.)
2. Complete heart block
3. 2 : 1 AV block
4. Atrial flutter or fibrillation with high degree of AV block
5. Sinus arrest with idionodal rhythm

Causes of sinus bradycardia
1. Congenital
2. Physical training
3. Convalescence from fever
4. Jaundice
5. Myxoedema
6. Hypothermia
7. Raised intra-cranial pressure
8. Drugs (digitalis)
9. Rapid rise in blood pressure
10. Transiently increased vagal tone (e.g. vomiting)

Further reading

Chamberlain, D. (1975) *Medicine,* 2nd. series, **25,** 1220

Causes of a 'dropped beat'
1. Sinoatrial block
2. Blocked atrial extrasystole
3. 2nd degree heart block

Causes of an irregular pulse
1. Extrasystoles (ventricular or supra-ventricular)
2. Atrial fibrillation
3. Sinus arrhythmia
4. Atrial flutter with varying block
5. 2nd degree heart block

Irregularity of volume also occurs in pulsus paradoxus and pulsus alternans

Causes of atrial fibrillation
1. Rheumatic heart disease, especially MS
2. Thyrotoxicosis
3. Myocardial ischaemia
4. Hypertension
5. Idiopathic ('lone') fibrillation, sick sinus syndrome or mitral valve prolapse
6. Chronic constrictive pericarditis
7. Atrial septal defect (over age 50)
8. Cardiomyopathy
9. Rarely atrial myxoma, bacterial endocarditis, acute pericarditis Ca bronchus, cor pulmonale, post-pneumonectomy, head injury

HEART BLOCK
Classification
1. Sinoatrial block
2. AV block
   1st degree, PR > 0.2 sec
   2nd degree
      (i) Dropped beats
         Fixed PR (Mobitz)
         Varying PR (Wenkebach)
      (ii) Fixed AV relationship (2 : 1, 3 : 1, etc.)
   3rd degree, Complete
3. Bundle branch block
4. Intraventricular block

Causes
1. Congenital (usually AV nodal)
2. Idiopathic
3. Ischaemic heart disease
4. Aortic stenosis
5. Drugs (digitalis)
6. Cardiomyopathy (including myocardial infiltration and collagen-vascular disease)
7. Myocarditis (rheumatic, diphtheritic)
8. Rarely trauma, tumour, syphilis, hypertension

Wolff-Parkinson-White syndrome (short PR, widened QRS with recurrent paroxysmal tachycardia) is due to congenital accessory pathway for AV conduction with premature ventricular activation

ARTERIAL HYPERTENSION

Causes of pulmonary hypertension
1. *Passive*
   Secondary to raised L atrial pressure (MS or LVF)
2. *Hyperdynamic*
   L to R shunt (ASD, VSD, PDA and TAPVD)
3. *Reactive*
      (i) Vasoconstriction secondary to hypoxia
            High altitude
            Chronic bronchitis
            Kyphoscoliosis
            Upper respiratory tract obstruction
            Respiratory depression
      (ii) Obstructive
            Pulmonary thrombi or emboli
            Arteritis
            Parasites, e.g. schistosomiasis

Causes of systemic hypertension

A *Essential*
B *Secondary*
   1. Renal
         (i) Ischaemia (esp. renal artery stenosis)
         (ii) Diffuse renal disease
   2. Hormonal
         (i) Phaeochromocytoma
         (ii) Cushing's
         (iii) Oral contraceptives (increase angiotensin precursor)
         (iv) Primary aldosteronism (Conn's)
         (v) Acromegaly
   3. Coarctation
   4. Polycythaemia vera
   5. Toxaemia of pregnancy
   6. Neurogenic e.g. head injury
   7. Acute intermittent porphyria
   8. ? Aortic valve homograft
   9. ? Alcoholism

CARDIOMYOPATHY
The definition varies but most authors exclude ischaemia (e.g. anaemia) and valvular disease (e.g. carcinoid). Note that hypertension is the only feature which distinguishes 'hypertensive heart disease with failure' from 'congestive cardiomyopathy'.

CAUSES

A. Primary
1. *Systolic pump failure*
      (i) Congestive cardiomyopathy (COCM)
      (ii) Endocardial fibroelastosis
2. *Diastolic compliance failure*
   Hypertrophic cardiomyopathy with or without obstruction (HOCM)
3. *Obliterative*
   Endomyocardial fibrosis

B. Secondary
1. *Infective*
      (i) Viral (post-myocarditis)
      (ii) Bacterial e.g. diphtheria toxin
      (iii) Protozoal e.g. schistosomiasis
                          toxoplasmosis
                          trypanosomiasis (Chagas')
2. *Metabolic and endocrine*
      (i) Pregnancy and puerperium
      (ii) Hyperthyroidism, hypothyroidism, hypoadrenalism, acromegaly
      (iii) Haemochromatosis, glycogen storage disease (Pompe's), gargoylism (Hurler's), porphyria
      (iv) Thiamine deficiency (beri-beri)
      (v) Amyloidosis
3. *Neuromuscular*
      (i) Muscular dystrophy, especially Duchenne's and dystrophia myotonica
      (ii) Friedreich's ataxia
4. *Vasculitis* (including Löffler's disease)
5. *Leukaemia or granulomatous infiltrate (sarcoidosis)*
6. *Allergic* e.g. serum sickness
7. *Drugs and chemicals*
      (i) Metals—cobalt, antimony, arsenic
      (ii) Alcohol
      (iii) Emetine
      (iv) Phenothiazine and tricyclic antidepressants
      (v) Anaesthetics
8. *Radiation*

Further reading
Goodwin, J.F. (1975) *Medicine,* 2nd series, **25,** 1286.

COMPLICATIONS OF MYOCARDIAL INFARCTION
1. Cardiac arrhythmia: Almost any, but particularly—
    (i) Sinus bradycardia often with nodal escape
    (ii) Supraventricular tachycardia, atrial flutter, atrial fibrillation
    (iii) Ventricular tachycardia, flutter or fibrillation
    (iv) Heart block (all degrees)
    (v) Cardiac asystole
2. LVF
3. Hypotension and 'shock'
4. Pulmonary embolism (usually from leg veins)
5. Mural thrombus and systemic emboli
6. Pericarditis
7. Ruptured papillary muscle (causing mitral regurgitation)
8. VSD
9. Cardiac aneurysm or rupture
10. Dressler's syndrome (with late onset pleuro-pericarditis)
11. Psychological, including 'L. chest pain'
12. Frozen shoulder and 'shoulder hand' syndrome
13. Iatrogenic; drugs, pacing, etc.

Further reading
Julian, D. (1975) *Medicine,* 2nd series, **29,** 1348.

Causes of generalised cardiomegaly on chest X-ray
1. Congestive cardiac failure
2. Multiple valve lesions
3. Pericardial effusion
4. Cardiomyopathy
5. Myocarditis
6. Ebstein's disease
7. Hyperdynamic circulation
8. Complete heart block

CAUSES OF SYNCOPE
(Transient loss of consciousness, usually due to inadequate cerebral blood flow or hypoxaemia)

1. Vasovagal
    (i) Emotion, heat, standing still
   (ii) Loss of blood or plasma, dehydration
  (iii) Carotid sinus hypersensitivity
  (iv) Postural hypotension
      Prolonged recumbency
      Vasodilator drugs
      Autonomic neuropathy: familial, diabetes, etc.
      Micturition syncope

2. Cardiac
     (i) Cardiac standstill-vagal inhibition
    (ii) Stokes-Adams (ht block)
   (iii) Ventricular tachycardia or fibrillation
   (iv) Aortic stenosis, HOCM
    (v) Cyanotic cong. ht. disease (fall in pO_2)
   (vi) Cough syncope (obstructed venous return)
  (vii) Massive pulmonary embolism
 (viii) Massive haemopericardium
   (ix) Atrial myxoma, ball-valve thrombus
    (x) Cardiogenic 'shock' (myocardial infarct)

3. Vascular defect
    (i) Carotid or vertebro-basilar insufficiency
      Atheroma, thrombosis, embolism
      Migraine
      Cervical spondylosis, strangulation, etc.
   (ii) Subclavian steal syndrome

4. Hypoxaemia
e.g., high altitude, anaemia
For other causes of coma, see p. 97.

CAUSES OF PERICARDITIS
1. Infective
   (i) Viral
   (ii) Bacterial (pyogenic or TB)
   (iii) Mycotic
   (iv) Parasitic
2. Rheumatic fever
3. Collagen-vascular, especially SLE
4. Myocardial infarct and Dressler's syndrome
5. Neoplasm, especially bronchial carcinoma
6. Uraemia
7. Trauma
8. Myxoedema
9. Drugs (phenylbutazone, procainamide, practalol)
10. Endomyocardial fibrosis (EMF)
11. Radiation
12. Idiopathic (probably viral)

Further reading
Hollman, A. (1975) *Medicine,* 2nd series, **29,** 1393.

CAUSES OF HYPERDYNAMIC CIRCULATION
1. Exercise or emotion (anxiety, fright, etc.)
2. Pregnancy
3. Anaemia
4. Pyrexia
5. Thyrotoxicosis
6. AV aneurysm
7. Paget's disease
8. Beri-beri
9. Hepatic failure
10. Hypercapnia
11. Erythroderma
12. Vasodilator drugs

ELECTROCARDIOGRAPHY
Cardiac axis

Leads with the maximum
positive deflection
indicate the cardiac axis

Normal axis is 0° to + 90°
Right axis deviation is + 90° to + 180°
Left axis deviation is 0° to – 120°
(But axis of 0° to – 30° may occur in stocky build, pregnancy and
ascites)

Ventricular hypertrophy

Minimal criteria for LVH
Either R in aVL > 13 mm.
Or R in V5 or 6 > 27 mm.
Or S in V1 + R in V5 or 6 > 35 mm., providing the circulation is not
hyperdynamic

Minimal criteria for RVH
Rs or qR complex in V1 or V3r with ventricular activation time
> 0.03 sec., QRS < 0.12 sec., and R axis deviation

Combined LVH and RVH
Signs of LVH in precordial leads with a frontal plane axis of more
than + 90°

ECG signs of infarction

1. *Antero-septal*
Pathological Q and/or ST elevation and T inversion in leads I, aVL and V1–4

2. *Antero-lateral*
Pathological Q and/or ST elevation and T inversion in leads, I, aVL and V4–6

3. *Inferior (diaphragmatic)*
Pathological Q and/or ST elevation and T inversion in leads II, III and aVF

4. *True posterior*
Tall R waves in leads V1 and V2. (Exclude RVH, RBBB and Wolff-Parkinson-White)

5. *Subendocardial*
ST depression and T inversion in overlying leads, with reciprocal ST elevation and upright T in leads from the opposite surface and in cavity leads

Causes of low T waves
1. Thick chest wall or emphysema
2. Pericardial effusion
3. Ischaemia
4. Myocarditis or cardiomyopathy
5. Constrictive pericarditis
6. Hypothyroidism, hypopituitarism or hypoadrenalism
7. Non-penetrating chest trauma
8. Drugs—digitalis, quinidine
9. Hypokalaemia or hypocalcaemia
10. Abdominal visceral disease e.g. pancreatitis, cholecystitis
11. Post-tachycardia
12. Physiological
    (i) Juvenile pattern (esp. in Negroes)
    (ii) Eating a large meal or swallowing ice
    (iii) Anxiety
    (iv) Delirium tremens
    (v) Hyperventilation

Further reading
Goldberg, M.J. (1975) *Advanced medicine Symposium 11,* ed. Lant, A.F. p. 322 London: Pitman.

Causes of LBBB
1. Ischaemic heart disease
2. Hypertension
3. Aortic valve disease
4. Cardiomyopathy
5. Myocarditis

Causes of RBBB
1. Normal (especially in young people)
2. RV strain (especially pulmonary embolism)
3. ASD (especially ostium secundum)
4. Myocardial ischaemia
5. Myocarditis

ECG changes of hyperkalaemia
Tall T
Prolonged PR
Flattened P
Wide QRS
May be ventricular tachycardia or fibrillation

ECG changes of hypokalaemia
Flattened T
Prolonged PR
Depressed ST
Tall U

Hypercalcaemia: shortens QT
HyPOcalcaemia: PrOlongs QT

Chest disease

LUNG ANATOMY
BRONCHO-PULMONARY SEGMENTS

Anterior

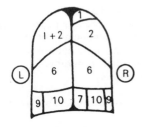

Posterior

Right lung
Upper lobe
  1. Apical
  2. Posterior
  3. Anterior

Middle lobe
  4. Lateral
  5. Medial

Lower lobe
  6. Apical
  7. Medial basal
  8. Anterior basal
  9. Lateral basal
  10. Posterior basal

Left lung
Upper lobe
  1 & 2. Apico-posterior
  3. Anterior
  4. Superior lingular
  5. Inferior lingular

Lower lobe
  6. Apical
  7 & 8. Antero-medial basal
  9. Lateral basal
  10. Posterior basal

LUNG MARKINGS

Upper border of lower lobe (oblique fissure). 2nd thoracic spine posteriorly to 6th rib in mammary line

Upper border of (R) middle lobe (transverse fissure). Horizontal line from 4th rib at sternum to the above line

Inferior border of lungs. 8th rib in mid-axillary line

PHYSIOLOGY
SPIROMETRY

The resting expiratory level is the most constant reference point on the spirometer tracing

Minute ventilation
Product of tidal volume and number of respirations per minute

Vital capacity
Largest volume a subject can expire after a single maximal inspiration. Normal values increase with size of subject and decrease with age (about 4½ litres in young adult male). Can be reduced in practically any lung or chest wall disease

Forced vital capacity (FVC)
The vital capacity when the expiration is performed as rapidly as possible

FEV$_1$ (Forced expiratory volume in one second)
Volume expired during first second of FVC

Ratio $\dfrac{FEV_1}{FVC}$ should be 75 per cent or more, and is reduced in obstructive airway diseases (asthma, emphysema, bronchitis)

Peak flow
Maximum expiratory flow rate achieved during a forced expiration. A convenient way to detect a reduction in ventilatory function. Also useful for serial measurements in the same patient and for assessing response to bronchial antispasmodics

Residual volume
Obtained by subtracting expiratory reserve volume from functional residual capacity. Residual volume is normally 20 to 25 per cent of total lung capacity but increases in elderly, and in over-inflation of the lungs (emphysema, asthma)

Anatomical dead space
The volume of air in the mouth, pharynx, trachea and bronchi up to the terminal bronchioles (about 150 ml). In disease the physiological dead space may greatly exceed the anatomical dead space due to disorders of the ventilation/perfusion ratio, but in health the two are identical

DIFFUSION
Rate depends on:
1. Pressure difference between alveolar gas and RBC
2. Thickness of tissue
3. Characteristics of tissue
4. Available surface area

Diffusion defects
Carbon dioxide is about 20 times more diffusible than oxygen. In diffusion defects the *arterial pO_2* is normal or slightly reduced at rest, but decreases markedly after exercise due to increased tissue uptake of O_2. *Arterial pCO_2* is normal or even reduced at rest (due to hyperventilation) and tends to fall on exercise

Diffusing capacity
Expressed as ml/min/mm Hg pressure difference (or mmol/min/kPa)
May be reduced in:
1. Alveolo-capillary block
    (i) pulmonary oedema
    (ii) pulmonary fibrosis
    (iii) infiltrative lesions, e.g. sarcoidosis and lymphangitis carcinomatosa
2. Reduction in area available for diffusion
    (i) emphysema
    (ii) multiple pulmonary emboli
    (iii) pneumonectomy, cysts, etc.
3. Anaemia
May be increased in:
1. Increased pulmonary capillary bed
2. Polycythaemia

Compliance
The volume change produced by unit change of pressure, expressed as litres/cm. H_2O (or l/kPa)

Pulmonary compliance
A measure of lung elasticity. It is reduced when the lungs are abnormally stiff due to pulmonary venous congestion or infiltrative or fibrotic lesions of the lungs. It is increased in emphysema

Thoracic cage compliance
Decreased in kypho-scoliosis, skeletal muscle spasticity and pectus excavatum

Further reading
Clarke, S. (1976) *British Journal of Hospital Medicine,* **15,** 137.
Saunders, K.B. (1975) *British Journal of Hospital Medicine,* **14,** 228.

Causes of hypoventilation
1. Respiratory centre depression
    (i) Drugs
    (ii) Anoxia
    (iii) Hypercapnia
    (iv) Trauma
    (v) Raised IC pressure
    (vi) Primary alveolar hypoventilation
        (Pickwickian syndrome, with obesity and hypoventilation)
2. Neural or neuromuscular cause
3. Respiratory muscle disease
4. Limited thoracic movement
    (i) Kyphoscoliosis
    (ii) Elevated diaphragm
5. Limited lung movement
    (i) Pleural effusion
    (ii) Pneumothorax
6. Lung disease
    (i) Obstruction in upper or lower respiratory tract
    (ii) Atelectasis, pneumonia, etc.

Causes of hyperventilation
1. Anxiety, hysteria, pain
2. CNS lesions: meningitis, encephalitis, trauma, CVA, etc.
3. Drugs: salicylates, analeptics, adrenaline
4. Increased metabolism: hyperthyroidism, fever, etc.
5. Anoxia
6. Metabolic acidosis
7. Pulmonary reflexes: Irritant gases, pneumothorax, atelectasis,
                        left ventricular failure
8. Hypotension
9. Artificial ventilation

PHYSICAL SIGNS
CRACKLES AND WHEEZES

Crackles
Crackles (formerly called râles, moist sounds or crepitations) are non-musical lung sounds of short duration. Inspiratory crackles are produced by abrupt opening of closed airways in regions of the lung deflated to residual volume. Early inspiratory crackles are associated with severe airways obstruction, late inspiratory crackles with a restrictive defect due to fibrosis, infiltration or oedema.

Friction between the two layers of the pleura can also produce crackles, but they are usually louder, localized and occur in expiration as well as inspiration.

Wheezes
Wheezes (formerly called rhonchi) are musical lung sounds produced by air passing at high velocity through an airway narrowed to the point of closure. The pitch of the wheeze is determined by the velocity of the air-jet and is independent of the calibre and length of the airway. Thus in severe airway obstruction wheeze may be absent if ventilation is so reduced that the air-jet slows below the critical minimum velocity.

Further reading
Forgacs, P. (1967) *Lancet,* **2**, 203.
Nath, A.R. & Capel, L.H. (1974) *Thorax,* **29**, 223.

COMMONLY CONFUSED SIGNS
Percussion

Skodaic resonance: hyperresonance above a pleural effusion level

Amphoric resonance: selective reinforcement of low-pitched vibrations by a cavity or pneumothorax

Cracked-pot sound: due to large cavity in communication with a bronchus

Vocal resonance

Whispering pectoriloquy: greatly increased vocal resonance, e.g. above a pleural effusion level

Aegophony: bleating sound heard occasionally above a pleural effusion level

Hippocratic succussion
Splashing noise due to gas and fluid in a cavity

Post-tussive suction
Sucking noise due to cavity springing open after a cough

EMPHYSEMA

Is characterised by enlargement of the air-spaces distal to the terminal bronchioles, either from dilatation or destruction of their walls. Some authorities (e.g. W.H.O. and American Thoracic Society) restrict the term to conditions accompanied by tissue destruction.

THE EMPHYSEMA—CHRONIC BRONCHITIS SPECTRUM

	Emphysema ('Pink Puffers')	Chronic Bronchitis ('Blue Bloaters')
Course	Relentlessly progressive dyspnoea	Intermittent dyspnoea with exacerbations
Sputum	Scanty	Profuse, mucopurulent
Cor pulmonale	Infrequent, usually terminal	Frequent and remittent
Polycythaemia	Uncommon	Common
CXR	Attenuated peripheral vessels	Normal peripheral vessels
Arterial pCO_2	Normal	Raised
Alveolar gas transfer	Reduced	Normal

CAUSES OF EMPHYSEMA

Localised
1. Congenital
2. Compensatory, due to lung collapse, scarring or resection
3. Partial bronchial occlusion
    (i) foreign body
    (ii) neoplasm
    (iii) peribronchial lymphadenopathy (e.g. TB)
4. Rarely unilateral emphysema due to bronchiolitis before age 8 years (Macleod's syndrome).

Generalised
1. Idiopathic ('Primary')
2. Associated with chronic bronchitis, chronic asthma or pneumoconiosis } usually centrilobular
3. Senile (physiological)
4. Familial (some due to α_1 anti-trypsin deficiency, when the disease is usually basal)

Further reading

Flenley, D.C. (1978) *Lancet,* **1,** 542
Hugh-Jones, P. (1973) *Advanced Medicine, 9th. Symposium,* ed. Walker, G. p. 300. London: Pitman.
Reid, L. (1975) *Hospital Update,* **1,** 115.

HARMFUL EFFECTS OF CIGARETTE SMOKING

1. *Pharmacological effects of nicotine*
   - (i) CVS: rise in BP, tachycardia, cutaneous vasoconstriction
   - (ii) Autonomic: transient stimulation, followed by depression of all ganglia
   - (iii) Adrenal: discharges adrenaline
   - (iv) CNS: stimulation, especially respiratory, vasomotor and emetic centres
   - (v) Antidiuretic: due to ADH release

2. *Pharyngeal and bronchial irritation*
   - (i) Bronchitis
   - (ii) Post-op. pneumonia, etc.

3. *Carcinoma incidence increased*
   - (i) Bronchus
   - (ii) Oesophagus
   - (iii) Prostate
   - (iv) Bladder

4. *Cardio-vascular disease exacerbated*
   - (i) Myocardial ischaemia
   - (ii) Buerger's

5. *Peptic ulcer mortality increased*
   (but *not* incidence)

6. *Idiosyncrasy*
   - (i) Tobacco angina
   - (ii) Atrial extrasystoles
   - (iii) Hypoglycaemia, etc.

7. *Tobacco amblyopia*
   (very rarely)

8. *Cirrhosis incidence increased*
   (probably due to associated alcoholism)

9. *Effect on fetus*
   Smoking during pregnancy restricts fetal growth and increases perinatal mortality rate

Further reading

Third Report of Royal College of Physicians of London (1977), 'Smoking or Health?' London: Pitman.

CAUSES OF CHRONIC COR PULMONALE

1. Chronic bronchitis or emphysema.
2. Chronic asthma.
3. Bronchiectasis.
4. Pulmonary fibrosis (p. 28)
5. Pulmonary thromboembolism.
6. Kyphoscoliosis.
7. Chronic neuromuscular disease affecting chest.
8. Primary alveolar hypoventilation (including Pickwickian syndrome).

Further reading

White, R. (1975) *Medicine,* 2nd series, **26,** 1336.

INDUSTRIAL CHEST DISEASE

1. *Mineral dust pneumoconiosis*
Coal dust, silicates (including talc, kaolin and asbestos), iron, tin, tungsten, aluminium, etc.

2. *Disease due to organic dust*
Byssinosis, farmer's lung, bagassosis, mushroom-worker's lung, paprika-splitter's lung, etc.

3. *Disease due to industrial gases and fumes*
Manganese pneumonitis, cadmium emphysema, silo-filler's disease, metal fume fever (ZnO), etc.

4. *Occupational lung cancer*
Nickel-refining, chromate workers, retort-house workers in gas-works, asbestos workers, etc.

5. *Chronic bronchitis.*
Many heavy, dusty industries

Further reading

Horne, N.W. (1976) *British Journal of Hospital Medicine,* **15,** 440.

CAUSES OF SLOW RESOLUTION OF PNEUMONIA

1. *Bronchial obstruction*
Neoplasm, foreign body (especially pea-nut), etc.

2. *Inappropriate chemotherapy*
Especially for staphylococcus, klebsiella, TB, mycosis

3. *Decreased host resistance*
Cachexia, agranulocytosis, immunoglobulin defects, LVF, etc.

4. *Pharyngeal pouch with 'spilling'*

5. *Formation of abscess, empyema or serous effusion*

6. *Other causes of pulmonary fibrosis* (p. 28)

CAUSES OF PULMONARY FIBROSIS

1. *Infections*
Especially TB, mycosis, varicella, psittacosis

2. *Pneumoconiosis*
Inorganic—
   Coal dust, silica, asbestos, talc, Be, Fe, Al, china-clay
Organic—
   Byssinosis, bagassosis

3. *Hypersensitivity*
Farmer's lung, bird-fancier's lung, pituitary snuff-taker's lung

4. *Fibrosing Alveolitis*
Including rheumatoid lung and desquamative interstitial
pneumonitis

5. *Aspiration*
Especially lipoid pneumonitis

6. *Cardiac*
Pulmonary oedema, mitral stenosis ossification, multiple pulmonary
infarcts, 'uraemic lung'

7. *Neoplastic*
Alveolar cell carcinoma, lymphangitis carcinomatosa

8. *Miscellaneous*
Sarcoidosis, systemic sclerosis, SLE, radiation, eosinophilic
granuloma, tuberose sclerosis (epiloia), xanthomatosis, biliary
cirrhosis, Paraquat poisoning, prolonged busulphan therapy

   When shown a chest radiograph with widespread miliary
densities do not offer pneumoconiosis as a first suggestion if breast
shadows are visible.

Further reading
Turner-Warwick, M. (1974), *British Medical Journal*, **2**, 371.
Scadding, J.G. (1974) *Thorax*, **29**, 271.

DRUG-INDUCED PULMONARY DISEASES

Drug	Pulmonary effect
1. Beta-blockers, aspirin, disodium cromoglycate	Asthma (pharmacological)
2. Many drugs, e.g. penicillin	Asthma (type I allergy)
3. Cytotoxics (esp. busulphan), ganglion-blockers	Fibrosing alveolitis
4. Pituitary snuff	Allergic alveolitis
5. Methotrexate	Granulomatous pneumonitis
6. Nitrofurantoin	Pulmonary eosinophilia with pleural effusion
7. Methysergide	Fibrosis and chronic pleural effusion
8. Procainamide, phenytoin, hydrallazine, isoniazid, etc.	Lupus erythematosus
9. Sulphonamides, etc.	Vasculitis
10. Heroin, methadone	Pulmonary oedema
11. Aminorex	Pulmonary hypertension
12. High conc. oxygen	Pneumonitis
13. Mineral oil (aspiration)	Pneumonitis or granuloma

Other drugs have indirect adverse effects on the lungs

1. *Infection* (esp. opportunistic or TB) due to glucocorticoids or cytotoxic drugs

2. *Aspiration* e.g. due to oversedation

3. *Pulmonary embolism* e.g. due to thrombophlebitis

4. *Bleeding* e.g. due to anticoagulants

Further reading
Davies, P. (1975) *Medicine,* 2nd series, **22,** 1074.
Rosenow, E.C. (1972) *Annals of Internal Medicine,* **77,** 977.

CAUSES OF LUNG ABSCESS

1. **Malignancy**
    (i) Necrotic bronchial carcinoma
    (ii) Secondary to bronchial obstruction
    (iii) Spill-over of pus or slough

2. **Aspiration**
    (i) Oral or pharyngeal sepsis
    (ii) Pharyngeal pouch
    (iii) Oesophageal obstruction, tracheo-oesophageal fistula
    (iv) Drowning
    (v) Bronchiectasis elsewhere in lung
    (vi) Coma, anaesthesia, alcoholic debauch, etc.

3. **Vascular embolus**
    (i) Secondary infection of pulmonary infarct
    (ii) Septic emboli due to pyaemia

4. **Specific Abscesses**
    (i) Staphylococcal
    (ii) Friedlander's (klebsiella)
    (iii) TB
    (iv) Actinomycosis and other fungi
    (v) Entamoeba histolytica

5. **Bronchial obstruction**
Benign tumour, foreign body, mucoviscidosis, etc.

6. **Infection of congenital or acquired cysts**

THE 'NORMAL' CHEST X-RAY

Faced in an exam. with a chest X-ray which at first sight appears normal, consider the following possibilities:
1. Small apical pneumothorax
2. Hiatus hernia behind the heart
3. Slight 'mitralisation' of the heart
4. Skeletal defects e.g. cervical rib
5. Secondary deposits in ribs or clavicles
6. Azygos lobe
7. Unilateral mastectomy
8. Gas under the diaphragm

CAUSES OF PNEUMOTHORAX

1. **Traumatic**
2. **Iatrogenic**
   (i) Thoracentesis, thoracic or cervical surgery
   (ii) Artificial pneumothorax
   (iii) Artificial ventilation
3. **Spontaneous**
   (i) *Localised air space disorder*
   Congenital bullae
   Localised emphysema
   Acquired cysts, etc.

   (ii) *Generalised emphysema*
   (iii) *Secondary to specific lung disease*
   Diffuse cystic disease
   e.g. congenital cysts, bronchiectasis, eosinophilic granuloma, tuberose sclerosis (epiloia)
   TB
   Silicosis
   Lung abscess
   Malignancy
   Hydatid cysts
   (iv) *Secondary to spontaneous mediastinal emphysema*
   Asthma, labour, straining at stool, etc.
   Rapid decompression of divers
   (v) *Associated with menstruation*
   ? Endometriosis

CAUSES OF PLEURAL EFFUSION

(A) *Transudate.* (Less than 2 g protein/100 ml fluid)
1. Cardiac failure
2. Nephrotic syndrome
3. Hepatic failure

(B) *Exudate.* (More than 2 g protein/100 ml fluid)
1. Pneumonia
2. Malignancy (bronchial Ca, secondary Ca, lymphoma or mesothelioma)
3. TB
4. Pulmonary infarction
5. Collagen-vascular disease (especially SLE)
6. Subphrenic abscess
7. Meig's syndrome (with ovarian fibroma)

Further reading
Emerson, P. (1975) *Medicine,* 2nd series, **23**, 1149.

CAUSES OF PULMONARY OEDEMA

1. **Increased capillary pressure**
   - (i) Left heart failure
     - Atrial e.g. mitral stenosis
     - Ventricular e.g. hypertension
     - or myocardial infarct
   - (ii) Pulmonary venous obstruction
   - (iii) Overload of i.v. fluid

2. **Increased capillary permeability**
   - (i) Pneumonia (viral, bacterial)
   - (ii) Inhaled toxins e.g. chlorine, mustard gas
   - (iii) Circulating toxins e.g. paraquat, septicaemia, snake venoms, histamine
   - (iv) Diffuse intravascular coagulation
   - (v) Renal failure
   - (vi) Radiation pneumonitis
   - (vii) 'Shock-lung' (post-traumatic)

3. **Decreased plasma oncotic pressure**
   Hypo-albuminaemia

4. **Lymphatic obstruction**

5. **Unknown mechanism**
   High altitude
   Raised intra-cranial pressure
   Heroin overdose
   Pulmonary embolism, esp. fat
   Eclampsia

Further reading

Flenley, D.C. (1974) *Advanced Medicine, Symposium 13,* ed., Ledingham J.G.G. p. 431. London: Pitman.

COMPLICATIONS OF CA. BRONCHUS
A. Local effects
1. Bronchial obstruction
    collapse
    pneumonia
    abscess
    emphysema
2. SV Caval obstruction
3. Pulmonary artery or vein compression
4. Cervical sympathetic, recurrent laryngeal or phrenic invasion
5. Pleural effusion, empyema
6. Direct spread into mediastinum, chest wall, brachial plexus, etc.
7. Erosion of large vessel

B. Metastases
Hilar nodes, liver, cerebrum, adrenals, bone

C. Non-metastatic extra-pulmonary effects
1. Cachexia, anaemia etc.
2. Hypertrophic pulmonary osteoarthropathy and clubbing
3. Neuropathy or myopathy (p. 110)
4. Skin lesions (p. 167)
5. Endocrine syndromes
    (i) Inappropriate ADH production
        Hyponatraemia
    (ii) Parathormone production
        Hypercalcaemia without radiological features
    (iii) Ectopic ACTH production
        Hypokalaemic alkalosis, weakness, oedema, diabetes
        mellitus and pigmentation
    (iv) Carcinoid syndrome
    (v) Pigmentation
    (vi) Thyrotoxicosis
    (vii) Hypoglycaemia
    (viii) Gynaecomastia
    (ix) Red cell aplasia

N.B. Polycythaemia very rarely occurs with bronchial carcinoma, but
may occur with renal carcinoma etc. (p. 139)

Further reading
Caplin, M. (1975) *Medicine,* 2nd series, **23,** 1135.
Ross, E.J. (1975) *Medicine,* 2nd series, **7,** 320.

HYPERTROPHIC OSTEOARTHROPATHY

A triad comprising
1. Clubbing
2. Periosteal new bone formation
3. Arthritis

CAUSES
1. **Thoracic**
   (i) Pulmonary neoplasm (Ca, mesothelioma)
   (ii) Chronic pulmonary suppuration
   (iii) Fibrosing alveolitis
   (iv) Mediastinal tumours, (p. 36)

2. **Cardio-vascular**
   (i) Bacterial endocarditis
   (ii) Cyanotic congenital heart disease
   (iii) Atrial myxoma
   (iv) Brachial arteriovenous fistula (unilateral)

3. **Extrathoracic lesions**
   (i) Gastro-enterological
       Cirrhosis (esp. biliary)
       Ulcerative colitis
       Crohn's disease
       Coeliac disease
   (ii) Thyrotoxicosis (thyroid acropachy)
   (iii) Rarely—Dysproteinaemia (esp. alpha chain disease)
              Pyelonephritis
              Syphilis
              Pregnancy

   4. **Congenital** *(Pachydermoperiostosis)*
      The syndrome may be only partially expressed, e.g. congenital clubbing

Possible pathogenetic factors
1. Increased levels of growth hormone and oestrogens
2. Increased autonomic activity (stimulation of afferent tracts of the vagus)
3. Increased circulating levels of reduced ferritin

Further reading
Katz, W.A. (1977) *Rheumatic Disease, Diagnosis and Management*, p. 676 Philadelphia: Lippincott.

Malignant tumours which metastasize to lung
1. Sarcomas
2. Bronchial Ca.
3. Breast Ca.
4. Renal Ca.
5. Thyroid Ca. } often clinically occult
6. Adrenal Ca.
7. Seminoma
8. Chorioepithelioma

Malignant tumours which metastasize to bone
1. Sarcomas
2. Bronchial Ca.
3. Breast Ca.
4. Prostatic Ca.
5. Renal Ca.
6. Thyroid Ca.
7. Neuroblastoma (in children)

CLINICAL FEATURES OF SARCOIDOSIS
1. Bilateral hilar lymphadenopathy (BHL)
   ↓
   BHL + pre-fibrotic pulmonary infiltration
   ↓
   Either resolution or pulmonary fibrosis
2. Constitutional symptoms, erythema nodosum, febrile arthralgia
3. Superficial lymphadenopathy
4. Skin lesions—lupus pernio, infiltrated plaques, nodules, infiltrates in scars
5. Ocular lesions—uveitis, conjunctival infiltrates, etc.
6. Neurological lesions
   (i) Neuropathy, especially facial nerve
       (Bilateral Cr. 7 LMN lesions strongly suggest sarcoidosis)
   (ii) Meningeal infiltration and local CNS deposits
7. Liver and spleen infiltration
8. Bone involvement, especially phalangeal cysts
9. Hypercalcaemia ± nephrocalcinosis and calculi
10. Nasal mucosal lesions
11. Uveitis, cranial nerve palsy, fever and parotitis (Uveo-parotid syndrome)
12. Rarely diabetes insipidus, GI lesions, etc.

MEDIASTINAL MASSES

Causes

1. *Lymphadenopathy*
   Lymphoma, sarcoidosis, infection (especially TB), carcinoma metastasis
2. *Aorta*
   Unfolding, aneurysm, coarctation
3. *Oesophagus*
   Corkscrew oesophagus (congenital elongation), mega-oesophagus (achalasia), enterogenous cyst, neoplasm
4. *Retrosternal goitre*
5. *Cysts*
   Dermoid, teratoma, pericardial 'spring-water' cysts, hydatid, bronchial cyst
6. *Thymoma*
7. *Herniae*
   Hiatus hernia, diaphragmatic herniae, lung herniation
8. *Neurogenic*
   Neurilemmoma, neurofibroma, sympathetic ganglioneuroma, sympathetic neuroblastoma
9. *Miscellaneous rare causes*
   Cardiac aneurysm or tumour, mesothelioma, lipoma, etc.

Further reading
Caplin, M. (1975) *Medicine* 2nd. series, **23**, 1148.

Common sites of mediastinal tumours

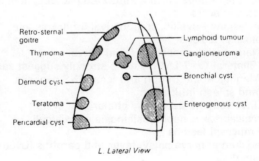

L. Lateral View

Gastroenterology

CAUSES OF DYSPHAGIA

1. **Mouth and pharynx**
   Stomatitis and glossitis
   Tonsillitis
   Quinsy, retro-pharyngeal abscess
   Lymphoma of tonsil

2. **Extrinsic compression of oesophagus or pharynx**
   Neck tumours
   Mediastinal tumours, glands, aneurysm, etc.
   Pericardial effusion
   Bronchial carcinoma

3. **Intrinsic disease of oesophagus or pharynx**
   Crico-pharyngeal achalasia
   Oesophageal achalasia
   Plummer-Vinson syndrome
   (Fe def., glossitis, pharyngeal web and koilonychia)
   Pharyngeal pouch
   Inflammation, stricture, or neoplasm
   Systemic sclerosis
   Chagas' disease (trypanosomiasis)

4. **Foreign body**
   Within the lumen of oesophagus or pharynx

5. **CNS lesions**
   Bulbar and pseudo-bulbar palsy
   Myasthenia gravis
   Diphtheritic neuritis

6. **Psychological (globus hystericus)**

Further reading
Atkinson, M. (1975) *Medicine,* 2nd series, **18,** 849.

CAUSES OF STOMATITIS

1. *Debilitation, smoking, alcoholism*

2. *Infection*
   (i) Viral
       Herpes simplex
       Herpangina
       Hand, foot and mouth disease
   (ii) Bacterial
       Pyorrhoea and alveolar abscess
       Vincent's angina, TB, Sy
   (iii) Fungal, especially Candida

3. *Associated with systemic disease*
   (i) Behcet's, Reiter's, Stevens-Johnson
   (ii) Leukaemia
   (iii) Neutropenia
   (iv) Fe deficiency
   (v) Vitamin deficiency
       B complex, including B_{12} and folate
   (vi) Cancrum oris (malnutrition, malaria etc.)

4. *Associated with skin disease*
   (i) Pemphigus vulgaris
   (ii) Benign pemphigoid of mucous membranes
   (iii) Lichen planus

5. *Stomatitis medicamentosa*
   (i) Cytotoxic drugs
   (ii) Bi, Hg, As, Au
   (iii) Antibiotics

6. *Aphthous ulcers*

7. *Leukoplakia*

8. *Neoplasm*

9. *Allergy*
   e.g. dentures and dental medicaments

10. *Caustics and trauma*
    e.g. cheek-biting and dentures

Systemic causes of gingival swelling
   1. Pregnancy and oral contraceptives
   2. Leukaemia (especially monocytic)
   3. Phenytoin
   4. Scurvy
   5. Heavy metals (especially Hg and As)

CAUSES OF VOMITING
1. **Feeding upsets (in infancy) and dietary indiscretions**

2. **GI irritation**
   Poisons
   Gastric ulcer
   Gastritis
   Enteritis

3. **Obstruction**
   Atresia
   Stricture (including malignancy)
   Stenosis
   Intussusception
   Volvulus
   Strangulated hernia
   Paralytic ileus

4. **Acute intra-abdominal inflammation**
   Hepatitis
   Pancreatitis
   Appendicitis
   Pyelonephritis
   Cholecystitis

5. **Metabolic and endocrine**
   Diabetic precoma
   Pregnancy
   Uraemia
   Hypoadrenalism

6. **CNS**
   Psychogenic
   Severe pain
   Drugs
   Migraine
   Motion sickness
   Meningitis
   Menière's, labyrinthitis
   Raised intra-cranial pressure

7. **Miscellaneous**
   Acute dilatation of stomach
   Cyclical vomiting
   Radiation sickness
   Pertussis, etc.

CAUSES OF PAROTID GLAND ENLARGEMENT

1. Infections
   (i) Viral (mumps, cytomegalic inclusion disease)
   (ii) Bacterial, especially in dehydrated patients

2. Neoplasia

3. Duct blockage
   e.g. by calculus

4. Systemic disease
   (i) Sjögren's syndrome
   (ii) Sarcoidosis
   (iii) Drugs (Iodides, thiouracil, phenylbutazone, lead)
   (iv) Cirrhosis
   (v) Cystic fibrosis
   (vi) Rarely—hyperlipidaemia, malnutrition or vitamin
      deficiency, pregnancy, diabetes mellitus

Further reading
Katz, W.A. (1977) *Rheumatic Disease. Diagnosis and Management*,
p. 211 Philadelphia: Lippincott.

CAUSES OF CONSTIPATION
ACUTE
1. *Ileus*
2. *Obstruction*
3. *'Simple' constipation* due to acute illness, hospital admission,
   travel, dehydration, low food intake, etc.
4. *Painful ano-rectal disease* e.g. fissure

CHRONIC
1. Disordered intestinal motility
   (i) *Small faecal residue* e.g. low fibre diet, dehydration
   (ii) *Over-use of purgatives*
   (iii) *Idiopathic bowel disorder*
      Irritable bowel syndrome (spastic colon)
      Idiopathic slow transit
      Idiopathic megabowel
   (iv) *Secondary to inflammatory bowel disease*
      e.g. diverticulitis,
      ulcerative colitis
   (v) *Metabolic*
      Early pregnancy
      Hypothyroidism
      Hypercalcaemia
      Hypokalaemia
      Acute intermittent porphyria
      Lead poisoning   *(contd.)*

(vi) *Drugs*
    Opiate derivatives
    Ganglion-blockers
    Anticholinergics
    Aluminium hydroxide
    Cholestyramine
    Iron salts
(vii) *Neuro-muscular disease*
    Spinal cord lesions
    Autonomic neuropathy
    Chagas' disease (toxic destruction of myenteric neurones)
    Systemic sclerosis (gut muscle degeneration)
    Hirschsprung's disease (genetic aganglionosis)
(viii) *Psychiatric*
    Depression, psychosis, anorexia nervosa, mental subnormality

2. **Obstruction**
Stricture, tumour, etc.

3. **Rectal dyschezia** (habitual neglect of call to stool)

Further reading
Hinton, J.M. (1972) *Management of Constipation*
ed., Avery-Jones, F & Godding, E.W. p. 79, Oxford: Blackwell.

CAUSES OF DIARRHOEA
ACUTE

1. **Dietary indiscretion** e.g. unripe fruit

2. **Food poisoning**
Animal
Plant
Bacterial (endotoxin or exotoxin)
Chemical

3. **Gastro-intestinal infection**
Viral
Bacterial
Protozoal
Helminthic

4. **Allergy**

5. **Psychogenic** (esp. anxiety)

(contd.)

CHRONIC

1. **Gastric**
   Gastrectomy
   Vagotomy
   Linitis plastica
   Pernicious anaemia

2. **Intestinal**
   Ulcerative colitis
   Crohn's disease
   Diverticular disease
   Neoplasm, etc.

3. **Malabsorption** (q.v.)

4. **Metabolic**
   Thyrotoxicosis
   Carcinoid
   Pellagra
   Medullary carcinoma of thyroid
   Tumour of APUD cells

5. **Drugs**
   e.g. purgatives

6. **Autonomic neuropathy**
   e.g. diabetes

7. **Spurious diarrhoea**
   (due to faecal impaction)

CAUSES OF MALABSORPTION

1. **Inadequate digestion**
   Gastric or intestinal resection
   Bile salt deficiency
   Pancreatic insufficiency (especially fibrocystic disease)
   Disorders of enterocyte brush border
   (i) Disaccharidase deficiency
   (ii) Enterokinase deficiency

2. **Parasites**
   Tapeworms
   Giardiasis, Strongyloides stercoralis, Diphyllobothrium latum
   Pneumatosis cystoidoses

3. **Change in intestinal bacterial flora** (p. 44)

4. **Intestinal hurry or fistulae**

5. **Enterocyte damage**
   Coeliac disease (Gluten intolerance)
   Cow's milk intolerance
   Soya flour intolerance
   Tropical sprue

6. **Infiltrative disorders**
   Crohn's disease
   Whipple's disease
   Lymphoma or leukaemia
   TB
   Systemic sclerosis
   Systemic mastocytosis
   Alpha-chain disease
   Amyloidosis

7. **Metabolic abnormality**
   Hartnup disease (malabsorption of neutral amino acids)
   Cystinuria (malabsorption of dibasic amino acids)
   Abetalipoproteinaemia
   Carcinoid
   Carcinomatous enteropathy
   Dermatogenic enteropathy (extensive eczema or psoriasis)

8. **Endocrine**
   Addison's hypoadrenalism
   Hypoparathyroidism
   Hyperthyroidism
   Medullary carcinoma of thyroid
   Zollinger-Ellison syndrome ⎱ (p. 137)
   Werner-Morrison syndrome ⎰
   Diabetes mellitus

9. **Vascular**
   Mesenteric arterial insufficiency
   Chronic venous congestion
   Lymphangiectasia

10. **Drugs**
    Liquid paraffin
    Neomycin, colchicine, cholestyramine etc.

11. **Radiation enteritis**

Further reading

Booth, C.C. (1973) *Topics in Gastroenterology* ed. Truelove, S.C. &
Jewell, D.P. Vol. I, p. 134, Oxford: Blackwell
Losowsky, M.S. (1975) *Medicine,* 2nd series, **18,** 874

CAUSES OF ABNORMAL GUT FLORA

1. **Abnormalities of gastric function**
    (i) Polya partial gastrectomy—Afferent loop syndrome
    (ii) Malfunctioning gastro-jejunostomy
    (iii) Pernicious anaemia

2. **Stasis**
    (i) Surgical blind loops
    (ii) Strictures
    (iii) Adhesions
    (iv) Small intestinal diverticulosis
    (v) Abnormal motility
        Systemic sclerosis
        Autonomic neuropathy
        Vagotomy
        Ganglion blocking agents
    (vi) Partial biliary obstruction with cholangitis

3. **Free communications between large and small bowel**
    (i) Gastrocolic fistula
    (ii) Enterocolic fistula
    (iii) Massive intestinal resection

Further reading

Tabaqchali, S. (1973) *Topics in Gastroenterology* ed. Truelove S.C. & Jewell, D.P. Vol. I, p.156. Oxford: Blackwell

CAUSES OF HEPATOMEGALY

1. **Raised venous pressure**
    Congestive cardiac failure
    Constrictive pericarditis
    Tricuspid stenosis
    Hepatic vein obstruction (Budd-Chiari)

2. **Degenerative**
    Fatty infiltration and early cirrhosis (esp. alcoholic)

3. **Myeloproliferative** (p. 78)

4. **Neoplastic**
    Primary (hepatoma, etc)
    Metastases
    Lymphoma

5. **Infective**
    Viral—Infective and serum hepatitis
           Infectious mononucleosis
    Bacterial —Hepatic abscess
                 TB, Syphilis
                 Brucellosis
                 Weil's disease
    Protozoal —Amoebic abscess
                 Malaria
                 Toxoplasmosis
                 Kala-azar
    Parasitic —Hydatid cyst

6. **Storage disorders**
    Amyloidosis
    Gaucher's
    Niemann-Pick's
    Histiocytosis X
    Glycogen storage disease
    Haemochromatosis
    Hurler's (gargoylism)

7. **Biliary obstruction**

8. **Congenital**
    Riedel's lobe (palpable, but not enlarged)
    Polycystic disease
    Congenital hepatic fibrosis

Causes of a hard knobbly liver
1. Carcinoma metastases
2. Cirrhosis with hepatoma
3. Polycystic liver
4. Hydatid cysts
5. Hepar lobatum (syphilis)

Causes of hepato-splenomegaly
1. Infective e.g. Infectious mononucleosis
2. Myeloproliferative, e.g. Myelofibrosis, chronic myeloid leukaemia
3. Some causes of portal hypertension, e.g. Budd-Chiari syndrome
4. Reticuloses
5. Storage diseases, e.g. Gaucher's disease, amyloidosis
6. Anaemia, e.g. PA, sickle-cell anaemia in children

CAUSES OF CIRRHOSIS

1. **Infection**
     (i) Viral hepatitis A and B
     (ii) ? Other viruses
     (iii) Congenital syphilis

2. **Toxins**
     (i) Alcohol
     (ii) Drugs e.g. methyldopa

3. **Prolonged cholestasis**
   e.g. biliary stricture

4. **Immunological**
     (i) Primary biliary (Hanot's)
     (ii) Active chronic hepatitis

5. **Metabolic**
     (i) Haemochromatosis
     (ii) Hepato-lenticular degeneration (Wilson's)
     (iii) Galactosaemia
     (iv) Fructosaemia
     (v) Glycogen storage disease
     (vi) Tyrosinosis
     (vii) Alpha-1-antitrypsin deficiency

6. **Venous stasis**
     (i) Prolonged congestive cardiac failure
     (ii) Hepatic vein occlusion

7. **Miscellaneous**
     (i) Cystic fibrosis
     (ii) Hereditary haemorrhagic telangiectasia (Osler's)
     (iii) Sickle-cell disease
     (iv) Jejuno-ileal bypass (for obesity)

8. **Idiopathic**

Further reading
Brunt, P.W. (1975) *Medicine,* 2nd series, **21**, 991.

PORTAL HYPERTENSION
CAUSES

1. **Extra-hepatic presinusoidal (Portal vein thrombosis)**
   Umbilical sepsis, exchange transfusion in neonates
   Suppurative pylephlebitis
   Portal lymphadenopathy (Ca. metastasis, lymphoma, etc)
   Clotting diathesis e.g. polycythaemia

2. **Intra-hepatic presinusoidal**
   Schistosomiasis
   Sarcoid, Hodgkin's, leukaemic infiltrates
   Congenital hepatic fibrosis

3. **Intra-hepatic postsinusoidal**
   Cirrhosis
   Veno-occlusive disease (Jamaican bush-tea)

4. **Extra-hepatic postsinusoidal**
   Hepatic vein obstruction (Budd-Chiari)
   Constrictive pericarditis, etc.

IDEAL CRITERIA FOR PORTA-CAVAL SHUNT
   1. Age under 40
   2. Portal vein patent
   3. Se Bilirubin $< 25 \ \mu$mol/l, Se Albumin > 30g/l
   4. No ascites
   5. No previous episodes of precoma
   6. Good nutrition
   7. High I.Q. not essential for patient's occupation

Complications of porta-caval shunts
   1. Operative risks
   2. Encephalopathy and myelopathy
   3. Hyperbilirubinaemia
   4. Gastric hyperacidity
   5. Haemochromatosis

HEPATIC ENCEPHALOPATHY

Cerebral dysfunction which can complicate all forms of liver disease and which particularly affects consciousness. The mean EEG frequency is slowed, nitrogenous substances are retained in the brain and giant astrocytes proliferate.

Clinical types of hepatic encephalopathy
1. *Chronic portasystemic encephalopathy*
2. *Cirrhosis with a precipitant*
   e.g.
      Diuresis
      Haemorrhage
      Paracentesis abdominis
      Diarrhoea and vomiting
      Surgery
      Alcohol
      Sedatives
      Infections
3. *Acute liver failure*
   e.g. due to
      Viral hepatitis
      Alcoholic hepatitis
      Drug reactions
      Paracetamol overdose

Factors affecting hepatic encephalopathy
1. Portasystemic collaterals
      (i) Extrahepatic e.g. varices, shunt
      (ii) Intrahepatic e.g. around cirrhotic nodules
2. Nitrogenous content of intestines
3. Bacterial action on colonic contents
4. Liver cell function

Further reading

Sherlock, Sheila. (1977) *British Journal of Hospital Medicine*, **17**, 144.

HEPATITIS
CLINICAL VARIANTS

Acute
1. Anicteric hepatitis
2. Classical acute hepatitis
3. Cholestatic hepatitis
4. Relapsing hepatitis
5. Fulminant hepatitis
6. Subacute hepatic necrosis

Chronic sequelae
1. Chronic persistent hepatitis
2. Active chronic hepatitis (q.v.)
.. Asymptomatic carrier state

Further reading

Sherlock, S. (1975) *Advanced Medicine, Symposium 11,* ed. Lant,
A.F., p. 72. London: Pitman
Woolf, I. & Williams, R. (1977) *British Journal of Hospital Medicine,*
17, 117

ACTIVE CHRONIC HEPATITIS *(formerly called 'lupoid hepatitis')*
A chronic disease, predominantly affecting the liver, with continuing
damage to hepatocytes and with evidence of abnormal
immunological activity.

Possible aetiological factors
1. Viral hepatitis
2. Drugs—Oxyphenisatin, methyldopa
3. Other chronic liver disease, especially alcoholic

Antibody reactions	% Positive cases			
	Active chronic hepatitis	Primary biliary cirrhosis	SLE	Control population
Anti-nuclear factor	65	40	>95	<5
Anti-mitochondrial	10	90	10	<1
Anti-smooth muscle	70	5	<1	3
Anti-glomerular	50	<1	<1	<1

Further reading

Joske, R.A. (1975) *Modern Trends in Gastroenterology.* ed. Read,
A.E. Vol. 5, p. 418. London: Butterworth.

LIVER TUMOURS

CAUSES OF PRIMARY LIVER TUMOURS

Hepatocellular Ca
1. Cirrhosis
2. Toxins
    (i) Aflatoxin (a metabolite of a mould which grows on rice and pea-nuts)
    (ii) Nitrosamines
3. Anabolic androgens
4. ? Poor nutrition

Cholangiocarcinoma
1. Parasitic infestation of biliary tree
    (i) Liver fluke—Clonorchis sinensis
    (ii) Schistosomiasis

Angiosarcoma
1. Previous 'Thorotrast' injection (for radiography)
2. Arsenic
3. Vinyl chloride monomer

Further reading

Terblanche, J. (1977) *British Journal of Hospital Medicine,* **17,** 103.

SOME 'METABOLIC' EFFECTS OF LIVER CELL CARCINOMA
1. Hypoglycaemia
2. Hypercalcaemia
3. Hyperlipidaemia
4. Hypertrophic pulmonary osteoarthropathy
5. Erythrocytosis
6. Dysfibrinogenaemia
7. Porphyria cutanea tarda
8. Carcinoid syndrome
9. Sexual precocity

Further reading

Murray-Lyon, I.M. (1975) *Medicine* 2nd Series, **21,** 1004.

ALPHA-FETOPROTEIN (AFP)

Occurs in plasma in:
1. Normal fetus
2. Elevated maternal AFP may indicate fetal neural-tube defect, twin pregnancy, intrauterine death, threatened abortion or subsequent low birth-weight
3. Hepatoma (in 90%)
4. Infective hepatitis, cirrhosis or liver metastases
5. Occasionally in primary Ca of stomach, ovary or testis

Occurs in increased conc. in amniotic fluid in:
1. Anencephaly
2. Open spina bifida
3. Omphalocoele
4. Bowel atresia
5. Turner syndrome
6. Congenital nephrosis
7. Intra-uterine death

Further reading

Harper, P.S. (1976) *Advanced Medicine Symposium 12,* ed. Peters, D.K. p. 457, London: Pitman.
Kew, M.C. (1975) *Modern Trends in Gastroenterology* ed. Read A.E. Vol. 5, p. 91 London: Butterworth.

HAEMOCHROMATOSIS

Haemosiderosis implies a pathological increase in tissue iron levels, but is not necessarily accompanied by cell damage

Haemochromatosis implies increased tissue iron with accompanying cell damage

Causes of haemochromatosis
1. *Primary* (dominant with incomplete penetrance)
2. *Secondary*
    (i) Multiple blood transfusions
    (ii) Inability to utilise iron
        a. Sideroblastic anaemia
        b. Thalassaemia
        c. Sickle-cell anaemia
    (iii) Increased iron ingestion (e.g. Kaffir beer made in iron cooking pots)
    (iv) Liver disease, especially due to alcohol
    (v) Porta-caval shunt
    (vi) Porphyria cutanea tarda
    (vii) Xanthinuria
    (viii) Congenital transferrin deficiency

Clinical features
1. Cirrhosis, often with hepatic pain
2. Skin pigmentation
3. Pancreatic insufficiency (exocrine and endocrine)
4. Testicular atrophy
5. Cardiomyopathy
6. Peripheral neuritis
7. Arthropathy (chondrocalcinosis)
8. Hepatic carcinoma is a complication

Further reading

Dymock, I.W. (1975) *Modern Trends in Gastroenterology* ed. Read, A. E. Vol. 5, p. 345. London: Butterworth.

HEPATO-LENTICULAR DEGENERATION (WILSON'S)
Clinical features
1. Cirrhosis
2. Neurological abnormalities: tremor, dysarthria, rigidity, intellectual deterioration
3. Kayser-Fleischer rings
4. Renal tubular defects: aminoaciduria, etc.
5. Osteomalacia, osteoarthrosis and osteochondritis
6. Cataracts
7. Blue lunulae of nails

LIVER DISEASE DUE TO DRUGS OR CHEMICALS

1. *Hepatic necrosis due to toxins*
   Halogenated hydrocarbons
   Heavy metals
   Iron or paracetamol overdose
2. *Hepatitis*
   Monoamine oxidase inhibitors
   Antidepressants
   Antirheumatic drugs
   Anticonvulsants
3. *Cholestasis*
   (i) Hypersensitivity e.g. chlorpromazine
   (ii) Steroid-cholestasis e.g. 17-methyltestosterone
4. *Generalised hypersensitivity* e.g. antibiotics
5. *Hepatic vein occlusion*
   Plant toxir s ('bush teas')
   Oral contraceptives
6. *Fibrosis or cirrhosis*
   Cytotoxins, especially methotrexate
7. *Interference with normal bilirubin pathway* (normal liver
   histology)
   (i) Haemolysis e.g. methyldopa
   (ii) Decreased uptake e.g. Filix mas
   (iii) Conjugation defect e.g. novobiocin
   (iv) Competition with bilirubin e.g. X-ray contrast media
   (v) Protein-binding release e.g. salicylates
8. *Hepatic hyperplasia, adenoma or carcinoma*
   Anabolic and androgenic steroids
   Oral contraceptives
   Nitrosamines
9. *Fibrosis or angiosarcoma*
   Arsenic
   Thorotrast
   Vinyl chloride

Further reading
Sherlock, Sheila. (1975) *Medicine,* 2nd series, **21**, 979.

MECHANISMS OF DRUG INTERACTIONS

1. *Interference with absorption*
   e.g. noradrenaline and local anaesthetics
   liquid paraffin and fat-soluble drugs
2. *Direct binding*
   e.g. chelating agents
3. *Competition at receptor sites*
   e.g. nalorphine and morphine
   anticholinergics and acetylcholine
4. *'Physiological' interactions*
   (i) Antagonists e.g. histamine and adrenaline
   (ii) Additives e.g. barbiturates and alcohol
   (iii) Potentiators e.g. digitalis and diuretics (hypokalaemia)
5. *Metabolism of drugs*
   e.g. phenobarbitone stimulates enzymes which catabolise other drugs such as phenytoin
6. *Protein-binding*
   Drugs bound by albumin may displace each other
   e.g. penicillin, sulphonamides, tolbutamide, phenylbutazone and warfarin

Further reading

Dollery, C.T. (1972) *Advanced Medicine* Symposium 8, ed. Neale, G. p. 185. London: Pitman.

FAMILIAL NON-HAEMOLYTIC JAUNDICE
Unconjugated
1. *Gilbert's*
   Decreased uptake of bilirubin by liver cell
   Mild intermittent jaundice
2. *Primary 'shunt' hyperbilirubinaemia*
   Increased production of bilirubin in marrow
   Very rare
3. *Crigler-Najjar*
   Hepatic glucuronyl-transferase deficiency
   Poor prognosis. Extremely rare
4. *Familial neonatal hyperbilirubinaemia*
   Glucuronyl-transferase inhibitor in serum
5. *Breast milk jaundice*
   Glucuronyl-transferase inhibitor in breast milk

Conjugated
1. *Dubin-Johnson*
   Mild intermittent jaundice
   Brown pigment in liver cells
   Characteristic BSP test with secondary rise at 2 hr. due to re-entry of conjugated bilirubin into blood
2. *Rotor*
   Similar but without hepatic pigmentation
3. *Summerskill and Walshe*
   Recurrent cholestasis of unknown cause

Further reading

Israel, J.B. & Arias, I.M. (1976) *Advances in Internal Medicine*, **21**, 77.

CAUSES OF HYPOCHLORHYDRIA
1. Pernicious anaemia
2. Gastric ulcer
3. Gastric carcinoma
4. Gastric polyposis
5. Subtotal gastrectomy
6. Iron deficiency
7. Pregnancy
8. Atrophic gastritis
9. Old age or debility
10. Vitamin deficiency (pellagra)
11. Radiation

CAUSES OF HAEMATEMESIS

1. Peptic ulcer
2. Oesophageal varices
3. Erosive gastritis (aspirin, alcohol, etc)
4. Hiatus hernia
5. Erosive oesophagitis
6. Mallory-Weiss syndrome (Oesophageal tear)
7. Blood dyscrasia
8. Gastric neoplasm
9. Haemorrhagic telangiectasia (Osler-Weber-Rendu)
10. Pseudoxanthoma elasticum
11. Ehlers-Danlos syndrome (Cutis hyperelastica)
12. Swallowed blood

PEPTIC ULCER

Indications for surgical treatment of peptic ulcer

1. Perforation
2. Continuous or intermittent bleeding
3. Pyloric stenosis
4. Suspicion of malignancy e.g. ulcer on greater curve, or positive cytology
5. Failure of medical treatment
6. Economic considerations and expediency
7. Serious persistent hour-glass deformity
8. Combined GU and DU
9. Very large ulcers
10. Gastric ulcer in patient over 60 with a short history

Side effects of vagotomy

1. Atony of stomach with dilatation
2. Belching and 'bilious' feeling
3. Abdominal distension
4. Diarrhoea
5. Cardiospasm

Medical complications of gastrectomy

1. Calorie deficiency
2. Stomal ulcer
3. 'Dumping syndrome'
4. Bilious vomiting, distension
5. Post-prandial diarrhoea
6. Malabsorption
7. Anaemia (deficiency of Fe, B_{12} or folate)
8. Osteomalacia
9. Hypoanabolic hypoproteinaemia
10. Increased risk of carcinoma in gastric remnant
11. Recrudescence of pulmonary TB

Further reading
Langman, M. & Alexander-Williams, J. (1975) *Medicine,* 2nd series, **18**, 863.

CAUSES OF CALCIFICATION ON ABDOMINAL X-RAY
1. Phleboliths
2. Calcified lymph nodes
3. Calculi (renal, gall-bladder, prostatic)
4. Calcified pancreas, adrenal, liver, kidney, aorta, psoas muscle, costal cartilage, etc.
5. Calcified tumour—dermoid, fibroid, etc.
6. Calcification in abdominal wall, e.g. cysticerci
7. Faecolith
8. Fetus

Further reading
Armstrong, P. (1976) *British Journal of Hospital Medicine,* **15,** 597.

CAUSES OF A MASS IN R. ILIAC FOSSA
1. Appendix abscess
2. Carcinoma caecum
3. Crohn's disease
4. Ileocaecal TB
5. Intussusception
6. Ovarian tumour, tubal pregnancy, etc.
7. Ectopic kidney
8. Actinomycosis
9. Carcinoid
10. Amoebiasis
11. Schistosomiasis

CAUSES OF ACUTE PANCREATITIS
1. **Biliary tract disease, including gall-stones**
2. **Alcohol**
3. **Idiopathic**
4. **Metabolic**
    (i) Hyperparathyroidism
    (ii) Hypercalcaemia
    (iii) Hyperlipidaemia
    (iv) Pregnancy and post-partum
5. **Trauma or surgery**
6. **Congenital defects**
    e.g. obstructed pancreatic duct
7. **Drugs**
    (i) Morphine
    (ii) Steroids
    (iii) Thiazide diuretics
8. **Viral**
    (i) Mumps
    (ii) Infectious hepatitis
    (iii) Infectious mononucleosis
9. **Parasitic**
    (i) Ascaris lumbricoides
    (ii) Clonorchis sinensis

10. Vascular disease
11. Carcinoma of pancreas
12. Hypothermia

Further reading

Waller, S.L. (1975) *Topics in Gastroenterology,* ed. Truelove, S.C. & Goodman, M. J. p. 97. Oxford: Blackwell.

CAUSES OF PROTEIN-LOSING GASTROENTEROPATHY

1. Giant gastric rugae (Ménétrier's)
2. Ulcerative colitis, Crohn's disease
3. Sprue
4. Intestinal lipodystrophy (Whipple's)
5. Malignancy, esp. gastric Ca.
6. Intestinal lymphangiectasia
7. Constrictive pericarditis, congestive cardiac failure
8. Hypogammaglobulinaemia
9. Erythroderma
10. 'Allergic gastroenteropathy' (? milk allergy)

MEDICAL CAUSES OF ACUTE ABDOMINAL PAIN

Some uncommon causes

1. Gastric dilatation, esp. in diabetic ketosis
2. Migraine
3. Epilepsy
4. Lead poisoning
5. Tabes dorsalis
6. Acute intermittent porphyria
7. Addison's disease
8. Haemochromatosis
9. Haemolytic crisis (especially sickle-cell anaemia)
10. Henoch-Schönlein purpura
11. Hepatoma
12. Hypercalcaemia
13. Uraemia
14. Intestinal parasites

COMPLICATIONS OF ULCERATIVE COLITIS

1. **Nutritional deficiencies**
   Anaemia
   Vitamin deficiency
   Dehydration
   Hypokalaemia
   Hypoproteinaemia
2. **Colonic**
   Acute toxic dilatation
   Perforation
   Massive bleeding
   Confluent crypt abscesses
   Carcinoma
   Stricture (in 10%, but rarely causes symptoms)
3. **Anal**
   Haemorrhoids
   Anal fissure
   Anal fistula
   Perianal abscess
4. **Ectodermal**
   Aphthous ulcers
   Clubbing
   Erythema nodosum
   Erythema multiforme
   Pyoderma gangrenosum
5. **Arthritis**
   Polyarthritis
   Sacro-iliitis
   Ankylosing spondylitis
6. **Ocular**
   Uveitis
   Episcleritis
   Keratitis
   Retinitis
   Retrobulbar neuritis
7. **Hepatic**
   Fatty infiltration
   Granulomata
   Focal necrosis
   Abscess (portal bacteraemia)
   Cirrhosis and chronic active hepatitis
   Pericholangitis
   Sclerosing cholangitis
   Rarely, biliary tract carcinoma

(contd.)

8. **Renal**
   Pyelonephritis
   Calculi
9. **Thrombo-phlebitis**
10. **Iatrogenic** (drugs, transfusions, surgery, etc.)

Further reading

Dyer, N. (1975) *Medicine* 2nd series, **19,** 898.
Sleisenger, M.H. & Fordtran, J.S. (1973) *Gastrointestinal Disease*
p. 1325 Philadelphia: Saunders.

COMPLICATIONS OF CROHN'S DISEASE

1. **Intestinal**
   Small bowel obstruction
   Fistulae, esp. into bladder, or vagina
   Perforation
   Suppuration and abscess formation
   Stricture
   Bleeding (usually slow, but may be massive)
2. **Ectodermal**
   Aphthous ulcers
   Clubbing
   Erythema nodosum
   Erythema multiforme
   Pyoderma gangrenosum
   Crohn's disease of mouth or skin (peri-anal or peri-ileostomy)
   Ectopic Crohn's of skin not contiguous to intestinal mucosa
3. **Nutritional deficiencies** (as for UC., p. 59)
   Due to
      (i) Decreased food intake
      (ii) Malabsorption—reduction in absorptive surface
                        disaccharidase deficiency
                        altered intestinal flora
                        intestinal hurry
      (iii) Loss of blood or protein into bowel
      (iv) Increased metabolic requirement
4. **Arthritis**
5. **Ocular**   } as for U.C. (p. 59)
6. **Renal**
7. **Amyloidosis** is commoner in Crohn's than in U.C.
8. **Hepatic complications** are less common in Crohn's than in
   U.C., but cholesterol gallstones occur

Further reading

Dyer, N. (1975) *Medicine,* 2nd series, **19,** 898.
Sleisenger, M.H. & Fordtran, J.S. (1973) *Gastrointestinal Disease,* p.
896 Philadelphia: Saunders.

CAUSES OF MULTIPLE INTESTINAL POLYPS
1. **Neoplastic**
   (i) Familial adenomatous polyposis coli
   Autosomal dominant
   Presents with diarrhoea
   Malignancy invariably develops
   Some patients have Gardner's syndrome (epidermoid cysts, osteomas, dentigerous cysts, lipomas, dermatofibromas)
2. **Hamartomatous**
   (i) 'Juvenile' polyposis coli
   Presents with prolapse or bleeding P.R.
   Not pre-malignant
   (ii) Peutz-Jeghers
   Peri-orificial lentiginosis with polyps mainly in small intestine
   Presents with anaemia or intussusception
   Very rarely associated with Ca. stomach or colon
3. **Inflammatory**
   Pseudo-polyposis
   Secondary to ulcerative colitis or colonic Crohn's
4. **Cronkhite-Canada syndrome**
   Generalised G.I. polyposis with alopecia, pigmentation and nail dystrophy. Very rare

Further reading
Bussey, M. J. R. (1970) *Gut,* **11,** 970.

COMPLICATIONS OF PARENTERAL NUTRITION
1. **Complications of central-vein catheterization**
   (i) Perforation of heart or blood vessel
   (ii) Thrombosis of vessel
   (iii) Air embolism
   (iv) Pneumothorax
   (v) Febrile reactions to pyrogens in tubing
   (vi) Infections, especially yeast or fungal
2. **Reactions to nutrients or lack of nutrients**
   (i) Allergic reaction
   (ii) Hyperosmolar syndrome with dehydration
   (iii) Hypoglycaemia on rapid cessation of glucose infusion
   (iv) Acidosis or liver dysfunction due to xylitol
   (v) Fluid overload and electrolyte inbalance
   (vi) Acne conglobata
   (vii) Deficiency states

Further reading
Law, D.H. (1972) *Advances in Internal Medicine,* **18,** 389.

CARCINO-EMBRYONIC ANTIGEN (CEA)

Occurs in plasma in:
1. Malignancy
     (i) endodermal adenocarcinoma (i.e. G.I. tract)
     (ii) bronchus, breast, neuroblastoma, female reproductive tract
          Higher values occur with poorly differentiated tumours,
          and after metastasis (over 100ng/ml)
2. Non-neoplastic disease of pancreas, liver or colon

Further reading
Brostoff, J. & Walker, G. (1975), *Immunology in Medical Practice* ed.
Taylor, G. p. 196 London: Saunders

GUT HORMONES

1. Gastrin
   Increased in
      i)   achlorhydria
      ii) after gastric surgery with bypass enterostomy.
      iii) some patients with DU
      iv) Zollinger-Ellison syndrome.
2. Secretin
3. Cholecystokinin-pancreozymin
4. Gastric inhibitory peptide (GIP)
5. Vasoactive intestinal peptide (VIP)
6. Motilin
7. Enteroglucagon (very high in dumping syndrome)
8. Somatostatin (from D cells of gut and pancreas)
9. Bulbogastrone, chymodenin, etc.

Further reading
Bloom S. (1975) *Medicine,* 2nd. series, **17, 818.**

Haematology

NORMAL VALUES IN HAEMATOLOGY

See note on SI units on p. 194
Imperial units are given in parentheses.

Haemoglobin
Men   13.5–18.0 g/dl (g. %)
Women 11.5–16.4 g/dl (g. %)

Red Cells
Men   4.5–6.5 × 10^{12}/l (4.5–6.5 million/c.mm)
Women 3.9–5.6 × 10^{12}/l (3.9–5.6 million/c.mm)

Haematocrit (PCV)
Men   0.40–0.54
Women 0.36–0.47

Mean cell volume (MCV)
Adults 76–96 fl(cμ)

Mean cell haemoglobin (MCH)
Adults 27–32 pg

Leucocytes
Adults 4–10 × 10^9/l. (4000–10000/c.mm)
Differential: Neutrophils 2500–7500 × 10^6/l
                    Lymphocytes 1500–3500 × 10^6/l
                    Monocytes   200–800 × 10^6/l
                    Eosinophils   40–440 × 10^6/l
                    Basophils   0–100 × 10^6/l

Platelets
150–400 × 10^9/l (150,000–400,000/c.mm)

Plasma viscosity
1.50–1.72 cp.

Parallels E.S.R. but is unaffected by age, sex or anaemia.

E.S.R. (Westergren)
Men–up to 5 mm/h.
Women–up to 7 mm/h

RED CELL SHAPE

Our understanding of changes of RBC shape has improved with the use of stereoscan electron microscopy (SEM)

Cell Types	Causes
1. Echinocyte ('Burr' cell)	1. Uraemia 2. Ca stomach or bleeding peptic ulcer 3. Post transfusion with old blood 4. Low-potassium red cells 5. Pyruvate kinase deficiency
2. Stomatocyte ('Mouth' cell)	1. Hereditary stomatocytosis 2. Liver disease 3. RBC sodium-pump defect
3. Codocyte ('Target' cell) 'Target' on dried film Bell shaped on SEM	1. Obstructive liver disease 2. Haemoglobinopathies 3. Thalassaemia 4. Iron deficiency 5. Post-splenectomy 6. L.C.A.T. deficiency
4. Acanthocyte ('Spur' cell)	1. Abetalipoproteinaemia 2. Alcoholic liver disease 3. Post-splenectomy 4. Malabsorption
5. Spherocyte ('Spherical' cell)	1. Hereditary spherocytosis 2. Immune haemolytic anaemia 3. Heinz body haemolytic anaemia 4. Post-transfusion 5. Water-dilution anaemia 6. Fragmentation haemolysis
6. Elliptocyte ('Oval' cell)	1. Hereditary elliptocytosis 2. Thalassaemia 3. Iron deficiency 4. Myelophthistic anaemia 5. Megaloblastic anaemia
7. Schizocyte ('Helmet' cell)	1. Microangiopathic haemolytic anaemia 2. Heart valve haemolysis (e.g. prosthesis) 3. Severe burns or calcification 4. March haemoglobinuria

8. **Drepanocyte** ('Sickle' cell)   Haemoglobinopathies, SS, S-trait, SC, etc.

   Varying spiculated shapes
   e.g. 'Sickle' or 'Holly-leaf'

9. **Dacryocyte** ('Teardrop' cell)   1. Myelofibrosis with myeloid metaplasia
                   2. Myelophthistic anaemia
                                       3. Thalassaemia

10. **Leptocyte** ('Wafer' cell)   1. Thalassaemia
                   2. Obstructive liver disease

N.B. Myelophthistic anaemia is due to a disrupted vascular pattern of the marrow. Causes include metastasis, lymphoma, myelofibrosis and T.B.

Further reading
Lessin, L.S., Klug P.P. & Jensen W.N. (1976) *Advances in Internal Medicine,* **21**, 451.

RBC abnormalities produced by absent spleen
1. Target cells
2. Acanthocytes
3. Schizocytes
4. Howell-Jolly bodies

RED CELL INCLUSION BODIES
Howell-Jolly bodies
Nuclear remnants seen as small dense purple particles at the periphery.

Causes
1. Splenectomy and splenic atrophy (p. 81)
2. Dyshaemopoietic states: leukaemia, megoblastic anaemia, etc.

Pappenheimer bodies
Fe-containing granules in siderocytes
Causes
1. Sideroblastic anaemia (p. 66)
2. Haemolytic anaemia, esp. after splenectomy

Heinz bodies
Occur in reticulocyte preparations as peripheral rounded dark blue bodies (globin denatured by oxidants)

Causes
1. Haemolytic anaemia due to oxidant drugs and chemicals
2. RBC enzyme defects, e.g. G6PD deficiency
3. Rare haemoglobinopathies ('unstable haemoglobins' e.g. Hb Koln) after splenectomy

HYPOCHROMIC ANAEMIA

Causes of hypochromic anaemia other than Fe deficiency
1. Infection
2. Rh. arthritis
3. Uraemia
4. Malignancy

} though more often normochromic

5. Thalassaemia major and minor
6. Sideroblastic anaemia (q.v.)

Causes of sideroblastic anaemia
(Defined as hypochromic anaemia with 'ring sideroblasts' in the marrow)
1. *Hereditary*
   Usually sex-linked. May or may not respond to pyridoxine
2. *Idiopathic*
3. *Drugs*
   (i) Alcohol
   (ii) Antituberculous drugs
   (iii) Chloramphenicol
4. *Lead poisoning*
5. *Myeloproliferative disease*
6. *Haemolytic anaemia*
7. *Miscellaneous non-haematological disorders*
   (i) Malabsorption
   (ii) Infections
   (iii) Collagen-vascular disease
   (iv) Cutaneous porphyria

Further reading

White, J.M. (1974) *Blood and its disorders* ed. Hardisty, R.M. & Weatherall, D.J. p. 808. Oxford: Blackwell.

Haematological effects of lead poisoning
1. Anaemia
2. Basophilic stippling
3. Reticulocytosis
4. Erythroid hyperplasia and 'ring sideroblasts' in marrow
5. Increased Se Fe in adults
6. 'Fast' Hb (on electrophoresis) in children with Fe deficiency

Further reading

White, J.M. (1974) *Blood and its disorders*, p. 821, ed. Hardisty, R.M. & Weatherall, D.J. Oxford: Blackwell.

HAEMOLYTIC ANAEMIA
CAUSES

1. **Congenital RBC defect**
   (i) Hereditary spherocytosis, elliptocytosis, stomatocytosis (p. 64).
   (ii) Hereditary non-spherocytic haemolytic anaemia
      Enzyme deficiency
      Thalassaemia (p. 69)
      Haemoglobinopathy, e.g. sickle-cell
      Idiopathic
   (iii) Acanthocytosis with abeta-lipoproteinaemia
2. **Acquired RBC defect**
   (i) Paroxysmal nocturnal haemoglobinuria
   (ii) Burns, radiation
   (iii) Secondary to RBC metabolic defect, e.g. megaloblastic anaemia or iron deficiency
   (iv) Secondary to other systemic disease, e.g. liver disease or vitamin E deficiency
   (v) Drugs and toxins (p. 68)
3. **Immune mechanisms**
   (i) Transfusion reactions
   (ii) Haemolytic disease of newborn
   (iii) Cold agglutinins (IgM, e.g. mycoplasmal pneumonia)
   (iv) Cold haemolysins (IgG, e.g. syphilis)
   (v) Autoantibodies (IgG)
      Idiopathic
      Leukaemia, lymphoma or carcinoma
      SLE or rheumatoid disease
   (vi) Drugs (p. 68)
4. **Infections**
   (i) Septicaemia
   (ii) Malaria (especially Blackwater fever)
   (iii) Bartonellosis (Oroya fever)
   (iv) Clostridium welchii
5. **Mechanical trauma**
   (i) Cardiac—openheart surgery, prosthetic valve, etc.
   (ii) Microangiopathic haemolytic anaemia (p. 68)
   (iii) March haemoglobinuria
6. **Hypersplenism**

CAUSES OF MICROANGIOPATHIC HAEMOLYTIC ANAEMIA (MHA)
1. 'Haemolytic uraemic syndrome' Thrombocytopenia, acute renal failure and MHA (usually in infants)
2. Thrombotic thrombocytopenic purpura (Moschowitz)
3. Renal cortical necrosis
4. Acute glomerulonephritis
5. Eclampsia, or post-partum
6. Malignant hypertension
7. Disseminated carcinomatosis
8. SLE or polyarteritis
In some cases the haemolysis is due to disseminated intravascular coagulation

Further reading
Gordon-Smith, E.C. (1974) *Blood and its disorders,* ed. Hardisty, R.M. & Weatherall, D.J. p. 763. Oxford: Blackwell.

HAEMOLYTIC ANAEMIA DUE TO DRUGS AND CHEMICALS
1. **Chemicals with direct toxicity**
    (i) Arsine, lead, chlorate, naphthalene
    (ii) Venoms, e.g. snake, spider
    (iii) Plant toxins, e.g. male fern
2. **Drugs with direct toxicity**
    Phenacetin abuse
3. **Drugs with an immunological effect**
    (i) Auto-immune (Antibodies directed against intrinsic R.B.C. antigens)
    Methyl-dopa
    Mefenamic acid
    (ii) Immune (Antibodies directed against the drug)
    Penicillin in large doses
    Cephalothin
    Quinidine
4. **Drugs acting on defective RBCs**
    (i) Hereditary enzymopathies (e.g. deficiency of G6PD, glutathione reductase, glutathione synthetase, etc.)
    Antimalarials, especially primaquine
    Sulphonamides
    Sulphones, especially dapsone
    Antipyretics
    Analgesics
    Nitrofurans
    Favism (broad beans)
    (ii) Unstable haemoglobinopathies (e.g. Hb Koln, Hb Zurich)

Further reading
De Gruchy, G.C., (1975) *Drug-induced blood disorders.* p. 156. Oxford: Blackwell
Pettit, J. & Hoffbrand, V. (1975) *Medicine,* 2nd series, **6,** 269.

Clinical manifestations of G6P Dehydrogenase deficiency
1. Drug-induced haemolysis
2. Infection-induced haemolysis
3. Broad bean-induced haemolysis (Favism)
4. Chronic non-spherocytic haemolysis
5. Neonatal jaundice (especially after Vit. K)

THALASSAEMIA SYNDROMES

A heterogeneous group of hereditary disorders characterised by decreased synthesis of either the α or the β chain of adult HbA ($\alpha2\beta2$).

Factors in the production of the anaemia
1. The Hb deficit produces a hypochromic microcytic anaemia
2. The relative excess of α or β chains precipitates in the red cell, forming inclusion bodies (Heinz bodies) which damage the RBC membrane and cause haemolysis
3. Folic acid deficiency
4. Mitochondrial iron deposition
5. Hypersplenism

Further reading
Forget, B.G. & Nathan, D.C. (1976) *Advances in Internal Medicine,* **21**, 97.

CAUSES OF MEGALOBLASTIC ANAEMIA
A) Folate deficiency
1. *Inadequate diet* (esp. alcoholics and old people)
2. *Malabsorption from upper intestine* (p. 42)
3. *Increased demand*
      (i) Infancy or pregnancy
     (ii) Increased cell turnover
           Myeloproliferative disease
           Malignancy or lymphoma
           Chronic haemolysis
           Chronic inflammation e.g. rheumatoid disease
4. *Anti-folate drugs*
      (i) Dihydrofolate reductase inhibitors
           Methotrexate, pyrimethamine, trimethoprim
     (ii) Impaired absorption
           Cholestyramine, sulphasalazine
    (iii) Uncertain mechanism
           Anticonvulsants, ethanol, oral contraceptives

(contd.)

B) Vitamin B$_{12}$ deficiency
1. *Malabsorption*
    (i) Lack of intrinsic factor
        Addisonian P.A.
        Partial or total gastrectomy
        Gastric atrophy due to gastritis
        Congenital P.A. with normal mucosa
        Rarely associated with polyendocrinopathy
    (ii) General malabsorption (p. 42)
    (iii) Specific B$_{12}$ malabsorption
        Ileal resection
        Ileal TB, Crohn's or ulcerative colitis
        Chelating agents (ingested phytates)
        Rarely congenital, with proteinuria
    (iv) B$_{12}$ utilisation by bacteria or parasites
        Blind-loop syndrome, diverticulosis, etc. (p. 44)
        Diphyllobothrium latum (fish tape-worm)
2. *Inadequate diet*
    Rare except in vegans and starvation
3. *Drugs*
    PAS, colchicine, neomycin, metformin

C) With normal folate and B$_{12}$
    (i) Cytotoxic drugs e.g. hydroxyurea, cytosine arabinoside
    (ii) Hereditary orotic aciduria (responds to uridine)
    (iii) Erythroleukaemia

Further reading
De Gruchy, G.C. (1975) *Drug-induced blood disorders.* p. 183
Oxford: Blackwell
Hoffbrand, A.V. (1975) *Advanced Medicine, Symposium 11.* ed. Lant,
A.F. p. 164 London: Pitman

Causes of macrocytic anaemia with normoblastic marrow:
1. Haemolysis $\left.\right\}$ since reticulocytes are macrocytes
2. Haemorrhage
3. Leukaemia
4. Aplastic anaemia
5. Marrow infiltration or replacement (q.v.)
6. Sideroblastic anaemia
7. Alcohol ingestion
8. Cirrhosis
9. Myxoedema or hypopituitarism
10. Protein deficiency
11. Scurvy

Causes of reduction in normal marrow activity
1. *Nutritional defect*
    (i) Fe, B_{12}, folate or pyridoxine deficiency
    (ii) Kwashiorkor
2. *Endocrine defect*
    (i) Erythropoietin deficiency (renal disease)
    (ii) Hypothyroidism
    (iii) Hypopituitarism
3. *Haemopoietic cell defect*
    (i) Aplastic anaemia (p. 72)
    (ii) Red-cell aplasia
4. *Marrow infiltration*
    (i) Myelofibrosis (and osteosclerosis)
    (ii) Malignant lymphoma
    (iii) Myelomatosis
    (iv) Metastatic carcinoma
    (v) Leukaemia
    (vi) Histiocytosis X
    (vii) Lipidoses (Gaucher's, Niemann-Pick's)
    (viii) Miliary TB

Further reading
Lewis, S.M. (1974) *Blood and its Disorders,* ed. Hardisty, R.M. &
Weatherall, D.J. p. 1113 Oxford: Blackwell

LEUCOPENIA

CAUSES OF NEUTROPENIA ($<2.5 \times 10^9$ neutrophils/l)
1. Pancytopenia (q.v.)
2. Infections
    (i) Viral
    (ii) Bacterial: typhoid, brucellosis, miliary TB,
            overwhelming septicaemia
    (iii) Rickettsial: typhus
    (iv) Protozoal: malaria, kala-azar
3. Drugs causing selective neutropenia: thiouracil, etc.
4. Megaloblastic anaemia
5. Hypothyroidism, thyrotoxicosis, hypopituitarism
6. Cirrhosis
7. Alcoholism
8. Idiopathic (chronic or periodic)

CAUSES OF PANCYTOPENIA
1. Aplastic anaemia (q.v.)
2. Acute leukaemia (in subleukaemic phase)
3. Marrow infiltration:
    (i) Malignant lymphoma
    (ii) Metastatic carcinoma
    (iii) Myelomatosis
    (iv) Myelosclerosis (in late stages)
4. Hypersplenism
5. Pernicious anaemia
6. SLE
7. Rarely disseminated TB

Types of aplastic anaemia

A. *With thrombocytopenia* (WCC may be low or normal)
1. Chronic acquired
    (i) Idiopathic
    (ii) Drugs or toxins
        Dose-related e.g. benzene, cytotoxics
        Idiosyncratic e.g. chloramphenicol, phenylbutazone
    (iii) Irradiation
2. Transient, following infection (especially hepatitis)
3. Congenital pancytopenia (Fanconi's)

N.B. (a) Pancytopenic aplastic anaemia may be complicated by
        paroxysmal nocturnal haemoglobinuria or leukaemia.
        (b) Chloramphenicol may produce either an early dose-related
        reversible marrow depression or, more rarely, an idiosyncratic
        severe aplastic anaemia of late onset.

(contd.)

B. *Red cell aplasia* (with normal WCC and platelets)
1. Chronic acquired
    (i) Idiopathic
    (ii) Immune, with thymoma and myasthenia gravis
2. Secondary to renal disease
3. Associated with haemolysis, infection or riboflavin deficiency
4. Congenital (Diamond-Blackfan)

LEUCOCYTOSIS
Causes of leucocytosis ($> 10 \times 10^9/l$ in adults)
1. Physiological
    (i) Infancy
    (ii) Pregnancy and post-partum
2. Infection
3. Haemorrhage
4. Trauma, burns, surgery
5. Myeloproliferative disease
6. Malignancy
7. Myocardial infarction and paroxysmal tachycardia
8. Drugs: steroids, digitalis, adrenaline
9. Chemicals: lead, mercury, carbon monoxide
10. 'Collagen vascular' disease
11. Metabolic disturbances: renal failure, gout, diabetic coma, eclampsia, etc.
12. Miscellaneous: haemolysis, Se. sickness, acute anoxia, spider venom, etc.

Causes of myeloid leukaemoid reaction (WCC $>50 \times 10^9/l$ or myelocytes or myeloblasts present in peripheral blood)
1. Infections, esp. in children and after splenectomy
2. Leuco-erythroblastic anaemia (q.v.)
3. Malignancy
4. Acute haemolysis

Causes of leuco-erythroblastic anaemia
1. Metastases to bone
2. Myelosclerosis
3. Myelomatosis
4. Malignant lymphoma
5. Marble bone disease (Albers-Schonberg)
6. Gaucher's, Niemann-Picks, Histiocytosis X

Causes of lymphocytosis ($> 3.5 \times 10^9$/l)
1. Infections
    (i) Viral: infectious mononucleosis; infective hepatitis;
        infectious lymphocytosis, influenza, exanthemata
    (ii) Bacterial: pyogenic infections in young children,
        convalescence from acute infections, pertussis,
        typhoid, brucellosis, TB, Sy.
    (iii) Protozoal: toxoplasmosis
2. Lymphatic leukaemia
3. Miscellaneous
    (i) Myasthenia gravis
    (ii) Thyrotoxicosis
    (iii) Hypopituitarism
    (iv) Carcinoma
    (v) Myelomatosis
4. Physiological in early childhood

Causes of eosinophilia ($> 440 \times 10^6$/l)
1. Allergy to food or drugs
2. Parasites: Hookworm, tapeworm, hydatid, ascaris, bilharzia,
   strongyloides, filaria, trichina, etc.
3. Skin disease
    (i) Scabies
    (ii) Dermatitis herpetiformis
    (iii) Atopic eczema
    (iv) Erythema neonatorum
4. Pulmonary eosinophilia
    (i) Asthma (including aspergillosis)
    (ii) Polyarteritis nodosa and variants (p. 159)
    (iii) Tropical eosinophilia
    (iv) Löffler's
5. Post-infectious rebound
6. Blood dyscrasias, including eosinophilic leukaemia
7. Malignancy, especially Hodgkin's
8. Eosinophilic granuloma
9. Post-splenectomy
10. Rheumatoid disease with extra-articular involvement

Causes of monocytosis ($> 800 \times 10^6$/l)
1. Infectious
   Viral—Infectious mononucleosis
   Rickettsial—Rocky Mountain spotted fever
   Bacterial—Listeria monocytogenes, TB, brucellosis, typhoid
   Protozoal—Malaria, kala-azar, trypanosomiasis
2. Hodgkin's disease
3. Monocytic leukaemia

HODGKIN'S DISEASE

The Rye classification
1. Lymphocytic predominance (Best prognosis)
2. Nodular sclerosis
3. Mixed cellularity
4. Lymphocytic depletion (Worst prognosis)

Essential criteria for the histological diagnosis of Hodgkin's disease
1. Complete or partial destruction of the nodal architecture (reticulin stain)
2. Presence of abnormal reticulum cells
3. Presence of Sternberg-Reed giant cells

Clinical Staging

Stage	Description
I	Disease limited to one anatomical region
II	(1) Disease limited to two contiguous anatomical regions on same side of the diaphragm
	(2) Disease in more than two anatomical regions or in two non-contiguous regions on same side of diaphragm
III	Disease on both sides of diaphragm but limited to involvement of lymph nodes, spleen and Waldeyer's ring
IV	Involvement of any tissue or organ other than lymph nodes, spleen or Waldeyer's ring

All stages are subclassified as A or B to indicate the absence or presence, respectively, of symptoms

Further reading
Harrison, C.V. (1975) *Recent advances in pathology* ed. Harrison, C.V. & Weinbren, K, **9**, 73. Edinburgh: Churchill Livingstone.

NON-HODGKIN'S LYMPHOMATA

Identification of more cell types in the lymph nodes has led to
increasingly complex classifications, but their relationship to
prognosis remains uncertain. The following classification
incorporates some of the newer concepts but avoids much of the
controversial terminology.

Bennett et al (1974)	Traditional name
A. *Follicular lymphoma*	
1. Cells predominantly small	
2. Mixed small and large cells	} Follicular lymphoma
3. Cells predominantly large	
B. *Diffuse lymphoma*	
1. Lymphocytic (i) Well-differentiated	
(ii) Intermediate	} Lympho-sarcoma
(iii) Poorly differentiated	
(iv) Mixed small and large	
cells	
2. 'Undifferentiated' large cell	} Reticulum cell sarcoma
3. Histiocytic (shown by E.M. and histochemistry)	
4. Plasma cell	} Plasmacytoma
C. *Unclassified*	

Further reading

Bennett, M.H., Farrer-Brown, G., Henry, K. & Jelliffe, A.M. (1974)
Lancet, **2**, 406.
Crowther, D., Scarffe J.H. (1977) Recent advances in medicine, ed.
Baron D.N., Compston N. & Dawson A.M., **17**, 41, Edinburgh:
Churchill Livingstone

CLASSIFICATION OF LEUKAEMIA

ACUTE (*'Poorly differentiated'*)

1. Acute myeloid (AML)
Subdivided according to predominant cells
    (i) Myeloblastic
    (ii) Promyelocytic
    (iii) Myelocytic
    (iv) Myelomonocytic
    (v) Monocytic
    (vi) Erythro-leukaemic

2. Acute lymphoblastic (ALL)
    (i) Null cell (80%)
    (ii) T cell
    (iii) B cell
Distinguished from other types by
    (i) peak incidence at 3-5 yr.
    (ii) better response to treatment, with long remission
    (iii) mature cells with normal morphology

CHRONIC (*'Well-differentiated'*)

1. Myeloid
    (i) Chronic granulocytic (CGL)
        Most are Philadelphia chromosome positive. In the atypical
        juvenile form, Hb F is increased
    (ii) Chronic myelomonocytic (with high neutrophil count)
    (iii) Chronic monocytic (with normal or low neutrophil count)
    (iv) Neutrophilic (very rare)

2. Lymphocytic
    (i) Chronic lymphocytic (CLL)
    (ii) Chronic leukaemia with lymphoma
        e.g. Waldenstrom's macroglobulinaemia
            Follicular lymphoma
            Diffuse lymphocytic lymphoma
            Sézary syndrome (with pruritus, erythroderma
            and Sézary T cells)

Further reading
Cawley, J.J. & Goldstone, A.H. (1975) *Hospital Update,* **1,** 719.

MYELOPROLIFERATIVE DISEASES

1. Primary polycythaemia vera
2. Myelofibrosis
3. Thrombocythaemia
4. Erythroleukaemia (Di Guglielmo)
5. Atypical myeloproliferative disorders

   Some authorities now exclude leukaemia from the myeloproliferative disorders, although transitions can occur as follows:

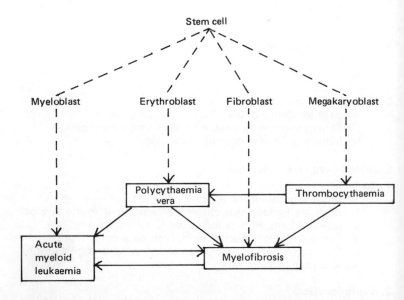

Further reading

Whitehouse, J.M. (1975) *Medicine,* 2nd series, **30**, 1687.

CAUSES OF POLYCYTHAEMIA

Absolute
1. Idiopathic PC Vera
2. Secondary
    (i) Hypoxic
        High altitude
        Cardiac or pulmonary disease
        Cerebral (decreased respiratory drive)
        Obesity (Pickwickian syndrome)
        Methaemoglobinaemia and sulphaemoglobinaemia
    (ii) Erythropoietin
        Kidney disease (p. 139)
        Carcinoma of liver
        Cerebellar haemangioblastoma
        Uterine myomata
        Virilizing syndromes
        Phaeochromocytoma
    (iii) Benign familial, due to abnormal Hb with either high
        oxygen affinity or excess methaemoglobin
    (iv) Hypertransfusion

Relative
1. Dehydration
2. 'Stress' polycythaemia (Gaisböck)
        Associated with hypertension, anxiety and high normal
        RBC mass or low normal plasma volume

Further reading

Wetherley-Mein, G. (1974) *Blood and its Disorders,* ed. by Hardisty,
R.M. & Weatherall, D.J. p. 1155, Oxford: Blackwell.

SPLENOMEGALY
Causes
1. Infections
   (i) Viral- infective hepatitis, infectious mononucleosis
   (ii) Bacterial: septicaemia, SABE, TB, Sy, brucellosis, typhoid
   (iii) Rickettsial: typhus
   (iv) Fungal: histoplasmosis
   (v) Protozoal: malaria, kala-azar, trypanosomiasis
   (vi) Parasitic: hydatid
2. Blood dyscrasia
   (i) Leukaemia
   (ii) Haemolytic anaemia
   (iii) Myelofibrosis
   (iv) Polycythaemia vera
   (v) Occasionally in ITP, myelomatosis, megaloblastic anaemia and chronic Fe-deficiency anaemia
3. Malignant lymphomas
4. Miscellaneous
   (i) Portal hypertension
   (ii) Lipoid storage disease
   (iii) Benign tumours and cysts
   (iv) Occasionally in SLE, sarcoidosis, amyloidosis, Rh. arthritis, hyperthyroidism, etc.

Causes of a huge spleen

Chronic myeloid leukaemia
Myelofibrosis
Malaria
Kala-azar
Gaucher's disease
Lymphocytic lymphoma

Look for evidence of iliac bone biopsy as this suggests myelofibrosis

Causes of moderately large spleen

Above 6
+ Storage diseases
  Haemolytic anaemias
  Portal hypertension
  Leukaemias

Causes of a just palpable spleen

Above 10
+ all other causes of splenomegaly (q.v.

HYPERSPLENISM

(reduction of 1 or more of the formed elements of the blood due to functional hyperactivity of the spleen)

Causes
1. Portal hypertension
2. Malignant lymphoma
3. Chronic lymphatic leukaemia or myelofibrosis, especially after repeated transfusions
4. Lipidoses (Gaucher's, Niemann-Pick's)
5. Sarcoidosis
6. Chronic infection
   T.B., brucellosis, bacterial endocarditis
   Kala-azar and malaria
7. Rheumatoid disease (especially Felty's syndrome)
8. Red cell disorders
   Congenital e.g. thalassaemia, spherocytosis
   Acquired e.g. auto-immune haemolysis, paroxysmal nocturnal haemoglobinuria
9. Idiopathic

Further reading

Richards, J.D.M. (1976) *British Journal of Hospital Medicine*, **15**, 505.

Common indications for splenectomy
1. Surgical, including trauma
2. Hereditary spherocytosis
3. Chronic ITP
4. Hypersplenism causing symptoms

Other indications
5. Acquired haemolytic anaemia
6. Acute ITP
7. Hereditary elliptocytosis
8. Myelofibrosis
9. Chronic lymphatic leukaemia
10. Malignant lymphomas
11. Thalassaemia major

ABSENCE OR ATROPHY OF SPLEEN

Causes
1. Splenectomy
2. Splenic infarct (including sickle cell disease)
3. Coeliac syndrome (including dermatitis herpetiformis)
4. Tropical sprue
5. Ulcerative colitis
6. Fanconi's anaemia
7. Congenital absence

PLATELETS

Causes of thrombocytopenia ($< 150 \times 10^9$/l)

1. *Decreased production*
    (i) Marrow aplasia e.g. drugs or toxins
    (ii) Marrow infiltration e.g. leukaemia
    (iii) Uraemia
    (iv) Megaloblastic anaemia
    (v) Alcoholism
2. *Decreased survival*
    Immunological
    (i) Idiopathic thrombocytopenic purpura (ITP)
    (ii) Drugs affecting platelets selectively e.g. quinine,
        sulphonamides, thiazides, rifampicin, indomethacin,
        phenylbutazone
    (iii) Blood transfusion with incompatible platelets
    (iv) 'Secondary' thrombocytopenia—
        a. SLE
        b. Chronic lymphatic leukaemia
        c. Auto-immune haemolytic anaemia with ITP
           (Evans' syndrome)
    Increased consumption
    (i) Disseminated intra-vascular coagulation (p. 89)
    (ii) Thrombotic thrombocytopenic purpura (Moschcowitz's)
    (iii) Large haemangiomata
    (iv) Infections—R.M. Spotted Fever
                    Typhus
                    Bacterial endocarditis
                    Meningococcal septicaemia
                    Exanthemata
3. *Sequestration*—Hypersplenism, hypothermia
4. *Dilution*—Massive transfusion of stored blood
5. *Loss*—Massive haemorrhage
In some conditions e.g. uraemia there may be several mechanisms
In neonates and children the following must also be considered:
1. Rare congenital disorders
    (i) Fanconi's aplastic anaemia (with multiple congenital
        anomalies)
    (ii) Familial thrombocytopenia
    (iii) Megakaryocyte aplasia
    (iv) Aldrich-Wiskott syndrome (with eczema and
         immunological deficiencies)
    (v) May Hegglin anomaly (with giant platelets)
2. Mothers with ITP, SLE or drug purpura
3. Viral infections: Congenital rubella syndrome
                     Toxoplasmosis
                     Cytomegalic inclusion disease
4. Cyanotic congenital heart disease
5. Haemolytic uraemic syndrome (p. 68)

Further reading
Sanderson, J.H. & Goldstone, A.H. (1977) *Hospital Update,* **3,** 249.

Causes of qualitative platelet defects (i.e. platelet dysfunction)

A. *Congenital*
  1. Hereditary thrombasthenia (Glanzmann)
      Impaired platelet aggregation
  2. Congenital abnormalities of platelet release or adhesion
  3. Giant platelet syndrome (Bernard-Soulier)
  4. Associated with other hereditary disease
      (i) von Willebrand's disease, and some haemophilia
      (ii) Hermansky-Pudlak (with albinism)
      (iii) Cutis hyperelastica (Ehlers-Danlos)
      (iv) Wiskott-Aldrich

B. *Acquired.*
  1. Drugs
      (i) Aspirin
      (ii) Indomethacin
      (iii) Phenylbutazone
      (iv) Streptokinase
      (v) High M.W. dextran infusion
  2. Systemic diseases
      (i) Uraemia
      (ii) Liver disease
      (iii) Dysproteinaemia
      (iv) Scurvy
      (v) SLE
  3. Myeloproliferative disease, esp. thrombocythaemia (excessive platelets of abnormal morphology)
  4. Aplastic anaemia or leukaemia

Further reading
Bowie, E.J.W. & Owen, C.A. (1977) *Recent advances in blood coagulation,* ed. Poller, L. No. 2, p. 59 Edinburgh: Churchill Livingstone.
Hellem, A.J. (1976) *Advances in Internal Medicine,* **17,** 171.

Tests of platelet dysfunction in thrombasthenia and von Willebrand's disease

	Thrombasthenia	von Willebrand's disease
Platelet aggregation		
1. To ADP	Absent	Normal
2. To collagen	Absent	Normal
3. To ristocetin	Absent	Absent
Platelet adhesion to glass beads	Low	Low or normal

Further reading
Brozovic, M. & Machin, S. (1977) *Hospital Update,* **3,** p. 203.

Causes of thrombocytosis (Increased platelets, $>400 \times 10^9/l$)
1. Haemorrhage, surgery, trauma
2. Splenectomy or splenic atrophy
3. Myeloproliferative disorders, especially megakaryocytic leukaemia and haemorrhagic thrombocythaemia
4. Chronic inflammatory disease
5. Malignancy
6. 'Rebound' after recovery from haemolysis or treatment of pernicious anaemia
7. Chronic renal disease

Further reading
Sanderson, J.H. & Goldstone, A.H. (1977) *Hospital Update,* **3,** 249.

Conditions predisposing to thrombosis

A. *Localised*
1. Stasis (tight bandages, etc.)
2. Damaged vessel wall
    (i) Infection
    (ii) Atheroma
    (iii) Trauma

B. *Generalised*
1. Thrombocytosis
2. Prolonged bed rest
3. Pregnancy and puerperium
4. Oral contraceptives
5. Hyperviscosity of blood (dysproteinaemia or polycythaemia)
6. Smoking
7. Congestive heart failure
8. Chronic infection
9. Blood group A1
10. Family history of thrombosis

Further reading
O'Brien, J.R. (1977) *Recent advances in blood coagulation* ed. Poller, L. No. 2, p. 241. Edinburgh: Churchill Livingstone.

VESSEL DEFECTS
Causes of bleeding due to defects of vessels or supportive tissues

A. *Acquired*
 1. *Vasculitis* (p. 159), especially Henoch-Schönlein purpura and allergic vasculitis due to drugs
 2. *Defect in connective tissue*
     (i) Senile purpura
     (ii) Cushing's disease or glucocorticoid therapy
     (iii) Scurvy (controversial, since platelets are defective)
 3. *Amyloidosis* (primary and secondary)
 4. *Anoxia*
     (i) Dysproteinaemia
     (ii) Fat embolism
 5. *Infections*
     (i) Bacterial endocarditis
     (ii) Septicaemia
     (iii) Viral and rickettsial infections
 6. *Dermatoses*
     (i) Eczema
     (ii) Pigmented purpuric dermatosis (Schamberg, etc.)
     (iii) Drug-induced capillaropathy, especially carbromal
     (iv) Simple easy bruising
     (v) Erythrocyte auto-sensitisation ('psychogenic' purpura)

B. *Congenital*
 1. Hereditary haemorrhagic telangiectasia
 2. Hereditary capillary fragility
 3. Pseudo-xanthoma elasticum
 4. Cutis hyperelastica (Ehlers-Danlos)

COAGULATION
The coagulation cascade

INTRINSIC

Collagen or
Kallikrein

$$XII \longrightarrow XI \longrightarrow IX$$

EXTRINSIC
VII

VIII, Ca^{++} and
phospholipid

X

V, Ca^{++} and
phosphilipid

Prothrombin ⟶ Thrombin

Fibrinogen ⟶ Fibrin

Ca^{++} XIII

Cross-linked
fibrin

Several new factors (Fletcher, Fitzgerald, Passovoy) involved in the
initial phase of intrinsic coagulation have been described, but their
role is not fully understood.
Factor XII is also involved in:
1. activation of fibrinolysis
2. conversion of kallikreinogen to kallikrein
3. formation of plasma permeability factor

Blood coagulation factors

I   Fibrinogen
II   Prothrombin
III   (Platelet lipid)
IV (Ca^{++})
V   Proaccelerin (labile)
VI   —
VII   Proconvertin (stable)
VIII   Anti-haemophilic globulin
IX   Christmas factor
X   Stuart-Prower
XI   Plasma—thromboplastin antecedent (PTA)
XII   Hageman
XIII   Fibrin-stabilising factor
Vitamin K deficiency affects II, VII, IX and X

Further reading

Baugh, R.F. & Hougie, C. (1977) *Recent Advances in Blood Coagulation* ed. Poller, L., No. 2, p. 1. Edinburgh: Churchill Livingstone.
Bowie, E.J.W. & Owen, C.A., (1977) *Recent Advances in Blood Coagulation,* ed. Poller, L. No. 2, p. 59. Edinburgh: Churchill Livingstone.

Factor VIII

Factor VIII has three components
1. VIII_c, necessary for coagulation, is measured by clotting assay
2. VIII_{vw}, necessary for platelet adhesion, is measured by ristocetin aggregation assay
3. VIII_{Ag}, which carries the active moieties, is measured by immunological assay

	Haemophilia A	von Willebrand's
VIII_c	Low	Low
VIII_{vw}	N	Low
VIII_{Ag}	N or High	N or Low

Platelets in von Willebrand's disease are probably not inherently defective, but only by virtue of the Factor VIII_{vw} deficiency

Further reading

Brozovic, M. & Machin S. (1977) *Hospital Update,* **3,** 203.
Sanderson, J.H. & Goldstone, A.H. (1977) *Hospital Update,* **3,** 249.

SCREENING TESTS FOR A BLEEDING DISORDER
1. **Blood count and film**
    To detect leukaemia and assess platelet number, size and shape
2. **Platelet count**
3. **Bleeding time** (with Duke's method, normal < 7 min.). Useful in diagnosis of von Willebrand's disease
4. **Hess test**, with sphygmomanometer cuff at c.100 mmHg for 5 min.
5. **One-stage prothrombin time** (N. 12–15 sec.)
    Tests the extrinsic system
    Prolonged in
        (i) Deficiency of II, V, VII or X
       (ii) Severe fibrinogen deficiency
      (iii) Presence of some inhibitors e.g. heparin or fibrin degradation products
6. **Activated partial thromboplastin time (APTT)**
    Tests the intrinsic system (especially VIII and IX)
    Uses kaolin in place of 'exposed collagen'
7. **Calcium thrombin time** (N. 10–20 sec.)
    Prolonged in
        (i) Fibrinogen deficiency
       (ii) Presence of some inhibitors, e.g. heparin
8. **Prothrombin consumption index**
    Very sensitive test which detects both platelet and coagulation abnormalities
9. **Fibrin degradation products**
    Increased in fibrinolysis
    Normal screening tests do not exclude vascular defects, e.g. senile purpura or mild coagulation factor deficiency, e.g. VIII (Haemophilia A) or IX (Haemophilia B)

Further reading
Brozovic, M. & Machin, S. (1977) *Hospital Update*, **3**, 203.

CAUSES OF FIBRINOGEN DEFICIENCY (< 1.5 g/l)
In many cases there are multiple causes.

Acquired
1. *Impaired formation* e.g. liver disease
2. *Increased consumption* ('disseminated intra-vascular coagulation', q.v.)
3. *Increased destruction* (excessive fibrinolysis)
   Usually secondary to 'disseminated intra-vascular coagulation'

Congenital
Very rare

DISSEMINATED INTRAVASCULAR COAGULATION
This is characterised by excessive formation of fibrinogen derivatives, usually due to increased proteolysis. There may be bleeding or thrombosis of any severity.

Causes
1. 'Shock', esp. Gram neg. septicaemia and anaphylaxis
2. Other infections, e.g. TB, viral and fungal
3. Obstetric
      Premature placental separation
      Retention of dead fetus
      Amniotic embolism
      Fetal death due to Rh incompatibility
4. Major surgery, especially with extra-corporeal shunts
5. Incompatible blood transfusion
6. Miscellaneous
      Leukaemia or carcinomatosis
      Liver, renal or prostatic disease
      Pulmonary embolism
      Snake venom

Minimum laboratory criteria for diagnosis
At least 2 of the following:
1. Increased fibrin degradation products in serum
2. Decreased plasma fibrinogen
3. Prolonged thrombin clotting time
4. Positive ethanol gelation
In severe cases there may be a decrease in platelets, and factors II, V and VIII

Further reading

Cash, J. (1977) *Recent Advances in Blood Coagulation* ed. Poller, L. No. 2, p. 293. Edinburgh: Churchill Livingstone.
Chesterman, C.N. (1975) *Advanced medicine, Symposium 11,* ed. Lant A.F. p. 191, London: Pitman

CAUSES OF HYPOPROTHROMBINAEMIA
1. *Vitamin K deficiency*
   (i) Dietary deficiency (uncommon)
   (ii) Defective synthesis by intestinal bacteria e.g. in neonates or after antibiotics
   (iii) Malabsorption e.g. biliary obstruction
   (iv) Renal failure (probably multifactorial)
2. *Liver disease*
3. *Drugs*
   (i) Vitamin K antagonists
   (ii) Thiouracil, salicylates, etc.
4. *Carcinomatosis* (uncommon)
5. *Congenital* (very rare)

Conditions associated with circulating anticoagulants
1. *Anticoagulants to AHG, etc.*
   (i) Haemophilia (? due to repeated transfusions)
   (ii) Pregnancy, often with Rh incompatibility
   (iii) Malignancy
   (iv) Collagen vascular disease
   (v) Pemphigus
   (vi) Idiopathic
2. *Heparin-like anticoagulants*
   (i) Irradiation
   (ii) Cytotoxic therapy

COMPLICATIONS OF BLOOD TRANSFUSION

1. *Febrile reactions*
    (i) Pyrogens
    (ii) Leucocyte or platelet iso-agglutinins
    (iii) Hypersensitivity to plasma
2. *Allergic reactions*
3. *Circulatory overload*
4. *Haemolysis.* Red cells of either donor or recipient may be affected
    (i) Blood group incompatibility
    (ii) Improper or overlong storage of donor blood
5. *Reaction due to infected stored blood*
6. *Disease transmission*
    (i) Se. hepatitis
    (ii) Syphilis
    (iii) Malaria
    (iv) Cytomegalovirus
    (v) Brucellosis
7. *Thrombophlebitis*
8. *Air embolism*
9. *Immunological sensitisation by compatible blood,* especially Rhesus sensitisation
10. *Transfusion siderosis*
11. *Complications of massive transfusion*
    (i) Collapse due to cold blood
    (ii) Excess citrate (exaggerates bleeding tendency)
    (iii) Excess ammonia from stored blood (exaggerates pre-coma in cirrhotics)
    (iv) Excess potassium (exaggerates hyperkalaemia in uraemic patients)
    (v) Thrombocytopenia
12. *Development of circulating anticoagulants* e.g. AHG antibody

Further reading
Tovey, G.H. & Bird, G.W.G. (1974) *Blood and its Disorders,* ed. Hardisty, R.M. & Weatherall, D.J. p. 1481 Oxford: Blackwell.

Neurology

Terms which are often confused

1. *Dysphasia.* Cortical disorder in use of symbols for communication, whether spoken, heard, written or read
Dysarthria. Disorder of articulation of speech
2. *Apraxia.* Inability to carry out purposive learned movements in absence of motor paralysis, sensory loss or ataxia
Agnosia. Failure to recognise, whether visual, auditory or tactile
3. *Perseveration.* Continuation or recurrence of an activity without appropriate stimulus
Verbigeration. Meaningless repetition of words or sentences
Echolalia. Parrot-like repetition by the subject of statements or acts made before them
4. *Epilepsy.* A paroxysmal transitory disturbance of brain function, ceasing spontaneously, with a tendency to recurrence
Myoclonus. A brief shock-like contraction of a number of muscle fibres, a whole muscle or several muscles, either simultaneously or successively
5. *Fibrillation.* Spontaneous contraction of individual muscle fibres (EMG finding)
Fasciculation. Spontaneous contraction of bundles of fibres in the same motor unit (seen clinically)
6. *Amaurosis.* Blindness from any cause
Amblyopia. Poor vision not due to retractive error or ocular disease
7. *Athetosis.* Involuntary slow coarse writhing movements, usually most pronounced in hand or arms
Dystonia. Involuntary sustained twisting movements, usually affecting proximal muscles

HARMFUL EFFECTS OF ALCOHOL (ethanol and congeners)
1. *Social complications of intoxication or alcoholism*
2. *Physical complications of acute intoxication*
   e.g. Accidents, coma, inhaled vomitus, Mallory-Weiss
        syndrome, 'hang-over'
3. *Neuro-psychiatric*
   (i) Withdrawal syndromes
       a. Tremulousness
       b. Psychoses (paranoia, hallucinations, etc.)
       c. Epilepsy (also pptd. by hypoglycaemia)
       d. Delirium tremens
   (ii) Nutritional deficiency syndromes
       a. Wernicke-Korsakoff syndrome
            Ophthalmoplegia with nystagmus
            Ataxia
            Confusion and dullness
            Amnesia and confabulation
       b. Peripheral neuropathy (Wallerian degeneration)
       c. Cerebellar degeneration
       d. Central pontine myelinolysis (produces bulbar palsy)
       e. Degeneration of corpus callosum
       f. Retrobulbar neuropathy ('alcoholic amblyopia')
   (iii) Toxic effects
       a. Acute myositis after a drinking bout
       b. Subacute myopathy (usually proximal)
   (iv) Neurological effects of liver disease
       a. Encephalopathy (p. 48)
       b. Myelopathy (esp. after porta-caval shunt)
       c. Neuropathy (mild but not rare)
   (v) Psychoses
            Paranoia, hallucinations, morbid jealousy, fugue,
            increased suicide risk, etc,
4. *Gastro-intestinal*
   (i) Acute gastritis and gastric ulcer
   (ii) Fatty liver or alcoholic hepatitis
   (iii) Cirrhosis
   (iv) Pancreatitis
   (v) Malabsorption
   (vi) Increased risk of Ca oesophagus
5. *Cardiac*
   (i) Arrhythmia
   (ii) Congestive cardiomyopathy
   (iii) Beri-beri heart disease
   (iv) Cardiomyopathy due to cobalt additives
6. *Haematological*
   Diminished haemopoiesis (RBCs, WBCs and platelets) due to
   dietary deficiency and toxic effect on marrow

(contd.)

7. *Metabolic*
    (i) Obesity or malnutrition
    (ii) Hypoglycaemia
    (iii) Hyperlipaemia
    (iv) Hyperuricaemia
    (v) Increased cortisol production
    (vi) Diuresis and electrolyte disturbance
    (vii) Haemochromatosis
    (viii) Porphyria cutanea tarda
8. *Increased incidence of infection,* esp. bacterial pneumonia, TB
9. *Effects on the fetus*
    (i) Increased risk of congenital defects
        a. Microcephaly
        b. Cardiac defect
        c. Growth deficiency
        d. Mental deficiency
    (ii) Increased peri-natal mortality

Further reading

Hore, B.D. et al. (1977) *British Journal of Hospital Medicine,* **18,** 106–143.

CAUSES OF DYSARTHRIA

1. *Bilateral upper motor-neurone (supranuclear) lesion of cranial nerves 9, 10 or 12 (Pseudo-bulbar palsy)*
    e.g. Cerebral ischaemia
          Motor neurone disease
          MS

2. *Lower motor-neurone lesion of cranial nerves 9, 10 or 12 (Bulbar palsy)*
    e.g. Motor neurone disease
          Bulbar polio
          Medullary tumour
          Syringobulbia
          Guillain-Barré

3. *Basal ganglion lesions*
    e.g. Parkinsonism
          Choreo-athetosis
          Hepato-lenticular degeneration (Wilson's)

4. *Cerebellar lesions*
    e.g. MS
          Toxins or drugs, especially alcohol
          Tumour

5. *Myasthenia gravis, facial muscular dystrophy and facial palsy*

6. *Oral lesions*
    e.g. False teeth
          Tongue-tie
          Cleft palate

CAUSES OF EPILEPSY

1. *Idiopathic (including genetic factors)*
2. *Focal lesions*
    (i) Birth injury
    (ii) Tumour esp. meningioma
    (iii) Trauma, scar
    (iv) Vascular
        Angiomatous malformation
        Cerebral ischaemia or infarct
        Acute hypertension
    (v) Infectious
        Encephalitis or meningitis
        Abscess or tuberculoma
        Neurosyphilis (p. 112)
        Hydatid or cysticercosis
    (vi) Primary dementias (p. 96)
    (vii) Other neurological disease
        Multiple sclerosis, leucodystrophies
        Tuberose sclerosis (epiloia)
3. *Metabolic*
    (i) Anoxia
    (ii) Hypoglycaemia
    (iii) Hypocalcaemia
    (iv) Alkalosis
    (v) Water intoxication
    (vi) Uraemia
    (vii) Hepatic coma
    (viii) Lipidoses (Tay-Sachs)
    (ix) Drugs and chemicals
        Nikethamide, lignocaine
        Lead poisoning
        Cocaine
        Ether
        Withdrawal of alcohol or barbiturates
    (x) Pyrexia, especially in children

CAUSES OF DISSEMINATED CNS LESIONS

1. Multiple sclerosis
2. Meningovascular syphilis
3. Multiple infarcts
4. Multiple metastases
5. Subacute combined degeneration
6. Tabes dorsalis
7. Friedreich's ataxia
8. Neuromyelitis optica
9. Diffuse sclerosis
10. Progressive multifocal leuco-encephalopathy

CAUSES OF DEMENTIA

Primary 'pre-senile' or 'senile' dementia
1. Idiopathic cerebral atrophy
2. Alzheimer's
3. Pick's
4. Creutzfeld-Jakob's transmissable dementia
5. Huntington's

Secondary
A. *Intra-cranial*
1. Tumour, especially frontal
2. Sub-dural haematoma
3. Vascular disease, esp. atheroma and multiple small infarcts due to thrombo-emboli from heart or large arteries
4. Trauma (includes repeated concussion of boxers and jockeys)
5. Infections
   (i) Encephalitis, abscess, meningitis
   (ii) Neuro-syphilis, esp. GPI
6. Multiple sclerosis and leucodystrophies
7. Neuro-lipidoses
8. Parkinsonism
9. Chronic epilepsy
10. Normal pressure hydrocephalus
11. Psychosis e.g. schizophrenia, chronic depression

B. *Extra-cranial*
1. Metabolic
   (i) Prolonged or recurrent anoxia or hypoglycaemia
   (ii) Chronic renal failure
   (iii) Hepatic failure
   (iv) Electrolyte imbalance
   (v) Carcinomatous neuropathy (p. 110)
2. Endocrine
   (i) Hypothyroidism
   (ii) Hypopituitarism
   (iii) Hypoadrenalism
   (iv) Hypo- or hyper-parathyroidism
3. Vitamin deficiency
   (i) B_{12} or folate
   (ii) Thiamine (esp. in alcoholics)
   (iii) Nicotinic acid (pellagra)
4. Drugs
   Barbiturates, cannabis, bromides, phenacetin
5. Toxins
   Alcohol, lead, manganese, arsenic, etc.

Further reading
Lishman, W.A. (1975) *Advanced Medicine Symposium 11,* ed. Lant, A.F. p. 128, London: Pitman.

CAUSES OF COMA
1. *Head injury*
2. *Epilepsy*
3. *Drugs*
    Alcohol
    Hypnotics
    Carbon monoxide
    Aspirin
4. *Metabolic*
    Hyper- or hypo-glycaemia
    Uraemia
    Myxoedema
    Hepatic failure
    Hypoadrenalism
    Hypopituitarism
    Hypocapnia
    Electrolyte imbalance
5. *Vascular*
    Cerebral thrombosis, embolism, haemorrhage
    Hypertensive encephalopathy
    Causes of syncope (p. 15)
6. *Pressure effects*
    Space-occupying lesions
    Hydrocephalus
7. *Acute infection of CNS*
    Meningitis
    Encephalitis
    Abscess
8. *Acute systemic infection*
    Malaria
    Septicaemia
9. *Hysteria or hypnosis*
10. *Hyper- or hypothermia.*

MECHANISMS OF HEADACHE PRODUCTION
1. *Skeletal muscle contraction* e.g. 'tension' headache
2. *Referred pain* e.g. disease of eyes, ears, sinuses, cervical spine
3. *Arterial dilatation*
    (i) Intra-cranial, e.g. systemic infections, hypertension, nitrites, anoxia, 'hang-over', post-ictal, concussion
    (ii) Extra-cranial, e.g. migraine
4. *Traction on arteries* e.g. raised IC pressure (haemorrhage, tumour, etc)
5. *Dilatation or traction on venous sinuses* e.g. post-lumbar puncture
6. *Inflammation*
    (i) Intra-cranial, e.g. meningitis
    (ii) Extra-cranial, e.g. giant-cell arteritis
7. *Psychogenic*

The Anatomy of the Facial Nerve

Causes of facial pain
1. Disease of teeth, sinuses, ear, nose or throat
2. Trigeminal neuralgia
3. Post-herpetic neuralgia
4. Aneurysm of post. communicating or int. carotid artery
5. Cranial arteritis
6. Migrainous neuralgia ('cluster' headache)
7. Raeder's paratrigeminal syndrome—Severe retro-orbital pain succeeded by ipsilateral miosis and ptosis
8. Superior orbital fissure syndrome—Boring retro-orbital pain and paresis of cranial nerves 3, 4, 5 and 6
9. 'Atypical facial pain'—Constant, nagging deep pain not corresponding to any anatomical sensory distribution
10. Temporo-mandibular arthritis
11. Myocardial ischaemia

Further reading

Graham, J.G. (1976) *Advanced Medicine, Symposium 12,* ed. Peters, D.K., p. 149 London: Pitman.

Ramsay-Hunt syndrome (geniculate herpes zoster)
1. Vesicles on auricle or anterior fauces
2. Pain in ear and mastoid region
3. Ipsilateral taste loss in anterior two-thirds tongue
4. Facial paresis or spasm
5. Deafness or dizziness
6. Hyperacusis (paralysis of n. to stapedius)

Causes of nystagmus
1. Physiological, e.g. opto-kinetic
2. Errors of refraction and macular lesions
3. Weakness of ocular muscles
4. Lesion of cranial nerves 3, 4 or 6
5. Brain stem lesions
6. Cerebellar lesions
7. Vestibular lesions
8. High cervical cord lesions
9. Idiopathic or congenital

Some causes of 'giddiness'
1. True vertigo (q.v.)
2. Hypotension or hypertension
3. Anaemia
4. Intra-cranial hypertension
5. Hypoglycaemia
6. Epileptic aura
7. Migraine
8. Psychogenic

Causes of vertigo
1. Vestibular lesions
    (i) Physiological
    (ii) Labyrinthitis
    (iii) Menière's
    (iv) Drugs, e.g. quinine, salicylates
    (v) Otitis media
    (vi) Motion sickness
    (vii) 'Benign post-traumatic positional vertigo'
2. Vestibular nerve lesions
    (i) Acoustic neuroma
    (ii) Drugs, e.g. streptomycin
    (iii) Vestibular neuronitis
3. Brain stem, cerebellar or temporal lobe lesions
    (i) Pontine infarction or haemorrhage
    (ii) Vertebro-basilar insufficiency
    (iii) Basilar artery migraine
    (iv) Disseminated sclerosis
    (v) Tumours
    (vi) Syringobulbia
    (vii) Temporal lobe epilepsy

BASAL ARTERIES OF THE BRAIN
Anatomy

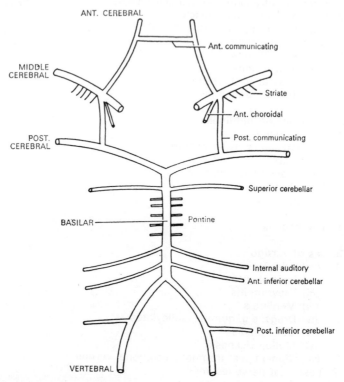

Features of post. inf. cerebellar artery thrombosis
1. Sudden onset of severe vertigo
2. Ipsilateral cerebellar ataxia, with nystagmus to side of lesion
3. Contralateral sensory loss of trunk and limbs to pain and temperature
4. Ipsilateral involvement of 5th to 8th nerves
5. Bulbar palsy
6. Ipsilateral cervical sympathetic paralysis

PATTERNS OF VISUAL FIELD LOSS

Causes of concentric diminution ('tunnel vision')
1. Glaucoma
2. Retinal disease, e.g. retinitis pigmentosa and choroido-retinitis
3. Papilloedema
4. Some types of optic atrophy, e.g. tabes dorsalis
5. Bilateral lesions of anterior calcarine cortex
6. Acute ischaemia e.g. migraine
7. Hysteria

Causes of central scotoma
1. Retinal disease involving macula
2. Retrobulbar neuritis (MS and Leber's optic atrophy)
3. Optic atrophy due to compression, toxins or B_{12} deficiency
4. Lesions of occipital pole (e.g. trauma)

Causes of bitemporal hemianopia
Central chiasmal lesions
1. Pituitary or peri-sellar tumour
2. Inflammatory, vascular or traumatic lesions

Binasal hemianopia
Very rare, being produced by bilateral lesions confined to the uncrossed optic fibres

Causes of homonymous hemianopia
Optic tract lesions—cerebral infarction or tumour may produce a hemianopia which bisects the macula.
Occipital cortex infarct

Causes of homonymous hemianopia with ipsilateral central scotoma
Lesions of lateral part of optic chiasma which also affect the optic nerve
1. Pituitary tumour
2. Aneurysm of ant. communicating artery
3. Sphenoidal wing meningioma

Causes of homonymous quadrantanopia
Anteriorly placed lesions of the optic radiation, especially temporal lobe tumours. More posterior lesions of the optic radiation become more hemianopic

CAUSES OF OPTIC ATROPHY

1. *Glaucoma*
2. *Retinal lesions*
   Choroido-retinitis
   Intra-ocular haemorrhage, etc.
3. *Optic neuritis* (retrobulbar neuritis) (q.v.)
4. *Chronic papilloedema*
5. *Pressure on optic nerve*
   Tumour
   Aneurysm
   Paget's disease
6. *Division of optic nerve*
   Surgery
   Trauma

CAUSES OF OPTIC NEURITIS

1. *Ischaemia* e.g. cranial arteritis
2. *Demyelinating disease*
   Multiple sclerosis
   Leucodystrophies
3. *Infective*
   Local: retinitis, periostitis, meningitis
   Systemic: syphilis, toxoplasmosis, typhoid fever
4. *Toxins*
   Methyl alcohol
   Lead
   Benzene
   Tobacco (defect in cyanide detoxication)
   Clioquinol (subacute myelo-optic neuropathy)
5. *Metabolic*
   Diabetes mellitus
   B_{12} deficiency
   Tropical ataxic neuropathy (cassava diet)
   Severe anaemia esp. haemorrhage
6. *Hereditary degenerations*
   e.g. Leber's, Friedreich's ataxia

CAUSES OF CATARACT

1. *Senility*
2. *Endocrine*
      Diabetes mellitus
      Hypoparathyroidism
      Corticosteroid therapy
      Cretinism
3. *Hereditary and congenital conditions*
      Rubella syndrome
      Atopic eczema
      Down's syndrome
      Hepatolenticular degeneration
      Galactosaemia
      Dystrophia myotonica
      Oculocerebrorenal syndrome (Lowe)
      Laurence-Moon-Biedl (retinitis pigmentosa, polydactyly, obesity, hypogonadism, mental retardation)
      Refsum's (retinitis pigmentosa, deafness, ataxia, neuropathy)
4. *Secondary to ocular disease*
      Glaucoma
      Ophthalmitis
      Degenerative myopia
      Retinal detachment
      Trauma
5. *Heat and irradiation*

CAUSES OF UVEITIS

(Uveal tract = iris, ciliary body and choroid)
1. *Miscellaneous systemic diseases*
      (i) Sarcoidosis
      (ii) Ankylosing spondylitis
      (iii) Ulcerative colitis
      (iv) Rheumatoid disease, esp. Still's
      (v) Reiter's disease
      (vi) Behcet's disease
2. *Infections*
      (i) Bacterial: TB
      (ii) Spirochaetal: Sy, relapsing fever, Weil's disease
      (iii) Protozoal: Malaria, toxoplasmosis
      (iv) Nematode larvae: Toxocara of dog and cat
3. *Secondary to ocular disease*
      (i) Ophthalmitis
      (ii) Trauma
4. *Idiopathic*

CAUSES OF PAPILLOEDEMA

1. *Raised intra-cranial pressure*
2. *Arterial hypertension*
3. *Optic neuritis* (papillitis)
4. *Obstructed retinal venous drainage*
     (i) tumour
     (ii) thrombosis of central retinal vein
     (iii) cavernous sinus thrombosis
5. *Miscellaneous rare causes*
     (i) Hypercapnia
     (ii) Exophthalmos
     (iii) SABE
     (iv) Hypoparathyroidism
     (v) Sudden or severe anaemia
     (vi) Vit. A poisoning
     (vii) Lead poisoning

Papilloedema without papillitis tends to produce a large blind spot but normal visual acuity
Papillitis (Retrobulbar neuritis) tends to produce a large central scotoma with poor visual acuity, and pain on eye movement

CERVICAL SYMPATHETIC PATHWAY TO THE EYE

1. Mid-brain (superior colliculus)
2. Tecto-spinal tract (adjacent to lateral spino-thalamic tract)
3. C8, T1 and 2 ventral roots
4. Cervical sympathetic trunk
5. Internal carotid and cavernous nerve plexus
6. Ophthalmic division of the trigeminal nerve

CAUSES OF PTOSIS

1. Congenital
2. Oculomotor nerve lesion
3. Cervical sympathetic lesion (Horner's)
4. Myasthenia gravis
5. Myopathy
6. Tabes dorsalis
7. Hysteria
Exclude congenital microphthalmos, contralateral exophthalmos

EYE MOVEMENTS

With the eye turned *laterally* the *elevators* and depressors are the *superior* and inferior recti respectively
With the eye turned *medially* the *elevators* and depressors are the *inferior* and superior obliques respectively

Causes of transient focal cerebral ischaemic attacks (TIA)
1. Emboli from heart or neck vessels
2. Mechanical effects
    (i) Cervical spondylosis
    (ii) Subclavian steal (proximal subclavian stenosis)
    (iii) Shunts
3. Increased arterial resistance e.g. hypertension or migraine
4. Hypotension
5. Increased blood viscosity e.g. polycythaemia
6. Anaemia

Further reading

Harrison, M.J.G. (1974) *Advanced Medicine, Symposium 10,* ed.
Ledingham J.G.G. p. 215. London: Pitman.

CAUSES OF RETINAL HAEMORRHAGE

1. Diabetes mellitus
2. Hypertension
3. Raised IC pressure
4. Retinal vein thrombosis
5. Trauma and retinal detachment
6. Arteritis (PN, cranial arteritis, etc.)
7. Sub-arachnoid haemorrhage
8. Severe anaemia, especially PA
9. Bleeding diathesis—defect in platelets (esp. leukaemia), vessels
   or coagulation factors

CAUSES OF SUDDEN BLINDNESS

1. Trauma—ocular or post-head injury
2. Vitreous haemorrhage, especially in diabetics
3. Retinal detachment
4. Acute glaucoma
5. Embolism of retinal artery
6. Thrombosis of retinal vein
7. Acute optic neuritis, esp. cranial arteritis and methyl alcohol
   poisoning
8. Cerebral infarct or haemorrhage
9. Hypertensive encephalopathy
10. Migraine
11. Acute hydrocephalus, esp. in children
12. Hysteria

SPINAL CORD
Transverse section

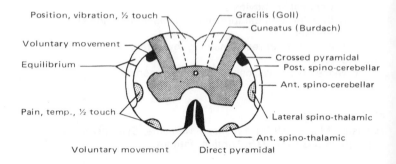

Tendon Reflexes

Ankle	S 1, 2
Knee	L 3, 4
Biceps	C 5
Supinator	C 5, 6
Triceps	C 7

Superficial Reflexes

Cremasteric	L 1, 2
Anal	S 3, 4
Plantar	S1
Abdominal	T 8 to 12

Nerve supply of diaphram
Phrenic n. (C 3, 4, 5) descends under cover of sternomastiod m., passes in front of subclavian artery, then descends vertically in front of root of lung and passes between pericardium and mediastinal pleura to diaphragm. The diaphragm is also innervated peripherally by the lower 7 intercostal nerves.

Course of recurrent laryngeal nerves
Right R.L.N. arises from vagus in the neck and winds backwards round first part of R. subclavian artery. *Left* R.L.N. arises from vagus in the superior mediastinum and winds backwards round arch of aorta. Both nerves then ascend between trachea and oesophagus and supply all muscles of larynx except cricothyroid.

    Bilateral paralysis causes stridor ('cadaveric' cords).

    Unilateral paralysis causes dysphonia with 'bovine' cough.

Causes of Cord Compression
1. *Vertebral*
    - (i) Congenital bony anomaly
    - (ii) Trauma
    - (iii) Vertebral collapse
    - (iv) Disc prolapse, spondylolisthesis, spondylosis
    - (v) Neoplasm (primary or secondary)
    - (vi) Paget's
    - (vii) Infection—TB or pyogenic
2. *Extra-dural*
    - (i) Hodgkin's, leukaemic infiltrate or metastases
    - (ii) Abscess
    - (iii) Cyst
3. *Intra-dural extra-medullary*
    - (i) Neoplasm (meningioma, neurofibroma)
    - (ii) Arachnoiditis
    - (iii) Arachnoid cyst
4. *Intra-medullary*
    - (i) Neoplasm, esp. glioma
    - (ii) Cyst or syringomyelia
    - (iii) Haematomyelia

Causes of paraplegia
1. Hereditary spastic paraplegia
2. Cerebral birth injury
3. Trauma
4. Cord compression—intra- or extra-medullary (q.v.)
5. Multiple sclerosis
6. Transverse myelitis
7. Spinal artery occlusion, including meningo-vascular Sy.
8. Syringomyelia
9. Motor neurone disease
10. Poliomyelitis
11. Sub-acute combined degeneration
12. Guillain-Barré (Landry's ascending paralysis)
13. Friedreich's ataxia; familial spastic paraplegia, etc.
14. Sagittal sinus thrombosis
15. Midline pre-central meningioma
16. Hysteria

PERIPHERAL NERVES
Nerve supply to muscles of front of forearm

Ulnar nerve supplies
1. Flexor carpi ulnaris
2. Half of flexor digitorum profundus

Median nerve supplies all the rest

Nerve supply to short muscles of hand

Median nerve supplies
1. Lateral two lumbricals
2. Opponens pollicis
3. Abductor pollicis brevis
4. Flexor pollicis brevis

Mnemonic—'Loaf'

Ulnar nerve supplies all the rest
Abductor pollicis brevis is paralysed in T1 root lesions but not in ulnar nerve lesions

To test abductor pollicis brevis the thumb is moved vertically against resistance, with the hand supine

Causes of wasting of small muscles of hand
1. Cord lesions at T1 level
    Motor neurone disease
    Tumour
    Syringomyelia
    Meningo-vascular Sy.
    Cord compression (p. 107)
2. Root lesions
    Cervical spondylosis
    Neurofibroma, etc.
3. Brachial plexus lesions
    Klumpke paralysis
    Cervical rib, etc.
4. Ulnar or median nerve lesions
5. Arthritis of hand or wrist, or disuse atrophy

Causes of Peripheral Neuropathy

1. *Idiopathic*
2. *Metabolic*
    Diabetes mellitus
    Amyloidosis
    Acute intermittent porphyria
    Chronic uraemia
    Dysproteinaemia
3. *Vitamin deficiency*
    Subacute combined degeneration (B_{12})
    B complex (alcoholism, beri-beri)
    Pellagra
4. *Infection*
    Diphtheria
    Leprosy
    Tetanus
    Botulism
5. *Drugs and Chemicals*
    Isoniazid, nitrofurantoin, vincristine
    Heavy metals (Pb, Hg)
    Organic chemicals e.g. triorthocresyl phosphate
6. *Miscellaneous*
    Collagen-vascular disease
    Malignancy (Lymphoma or Ca.)
    Sarcoidosis
    Guillain-Barré
    'Brachial neuritis' (Neuralgic amyotrophy)
7. *Mechanical*
    Trauma, compression, stretching
8. *Hereditary*
    Hereditary ataxias
    Hereditary sensory radicular neuropathy (Denny-Brown)
    Hypertrophic interstitial neuritis (Déjerine-Sottas)
    Peroneal muscular atrophy (Charcot-Marie-Tooth)
    Refsum's disease

Causes of mononeuritis multiplex
1. Polyarteritis nodosa
2. Diabetes mellitus
3. Leprosy
4. Carcinoma
5. Sarcoidosis
6. Rheumatoid disease

Types of non-metastatic carcinomatous neuromyopathy
1. *Encephalopathy*
   (i) Progressive multifocal leukoencephalopathy
   (ii) Polio-encephalopathy
   (iii) Cerebellar degeneration
   (iv) Dementia
2. *Encephalomyelitis*
3. *Neuropathy*
   Motor, sensory or mixed
4. *Neuromuscular disorder*
   (i) Myasthenia gravis
   (ii) Eaton Lambert syndrome (weakness which improves with tetanic stimulation)
5. *Dermatomyositis or polymyositis*
6. *Non-specific muscle wasting*

Dermatomes in the upper limb

Dermatomes in the lower limb

Dermatomes of head and neck

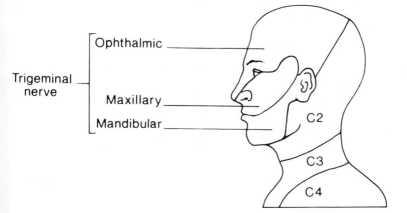

CLINICAL VARIETIES OF NEURO-SYPHILIS

1. Asymptomatic; Argyll Robertson pupils may be the only sign
2. Meningitis
     (i) Acute
     (ii) Chronic pachymeningitis
3. Vascular
     (i) Endarteritis of middle cerebral artery
     (ii) Endarteritis of anterior spinal artery (Erb's paraplegia)
4. GPI
5. Tabes dorsalis
6. Optic atrophy
7. Gumma of brain

Causes of absent knee and ankle jerks with an extensor plantar response

1. Sub-acute combined degeneration
2. Syphilitic tabo-paresis
3. Friedreich's ataxia
4. Motor neurone disease
5. Diabetes mellitus
6. Conus medullaris lesion

ARGYLL ROBERTSON PUPILS (ACCOMMODATION REFLEX PRESENT)

The light reflex is interrupted between the lateral geniculate body and the oculomotor nucleus (probably in the pre-tectal area)

Causes

1. Syphilis, esp. tabes dorsalis
2. Diabetes mellitus
3. Rarely alcoholism, encephalitis, MS or vascular or neoplastic lesions of midbrain

CAUSES OF A CHARCOT JOINT

1. Tabes dorsalis
2. Syringomyelia
3. Diabetes mellitus
Rarely:
4. Cord lesion e.g. trauma, meningomyelocoele, SACD
5. Leprosy, yaws
6. Congenital neuropathy (p. 109)
7. Congenital indifference to pain
8. Familial dysautonomia (Riley-Day)
9. Repeated intra-articular steroid injection

CAUSES OF TREMOR
1. Parkinsonism (q.v.)
2. Cerebellar lesion
3. Anxiety
4. Thyrotoxicosis
5. Alcoholism
6. Drugs e.g. tricyclic antidepressants
7. Heavy metals (e.g. 'hatters' shakes' due to mercury)
8. Neurosyphilis
9. Benign essential or familial tremor

CAUSES OF PARKINSONISM
(Tremor, rigidity and hypokinesia)
1. Idiopathic 'paralysis agitans'
2. Drugs—phenothiazines
            haloperidol
            reserpine
            methyldopa
            tetrabenazine
3. Toxins—manganese
            carbon monoxide
            kernicterus
4. Post-encephalitic
5. Repeated head injury
6. Rarely syphilis, cerebral tumour, hypoparathyroidism or
   Behcet's
Parkinsonian features also occur in
1. Phenylketonuria
2. Hepatolenticular degeneration
3. Shy-Drager syndrome (with autonomic dysfunction)
4. Progressive supranuclear palsy with paralysis of conjugate gaze
   (Steele-Richardson syndrome)
5. Creutzfeld-Jakob transmissible dementia
6. Olivopontocerebellar atrophy
Atheroma as a cause of parkinsonism is disputed

CAUSES OF DISORDERED NEUROMUSCULAR TRANSMISSION

1. *Hereditary*
    (i) Hereditary myasthenia gravis
    (ii) Pseudocholinesterase deficiency (suxamethonium paralysis)
2. *Drugs and toxins*
    (i) Depolarizing drugs
    (ii) Anticholinesterase poisons (e.g. 'nerve gas')
    (iii) Botulism
    (iv) Venom of Black Widow spider, puff-fish, etc.
    (v) Magnesium poisoning
    (vi) Antibiotics, especially Kanamycin
3. *Idiopathic myasthenia gravis*
    (possibly auto-immune)
4. *Myasthenia associated with other disease*
    (i) Thyrotoxicosis
    (ii) Malignancy (Eaton Lambert syndrome)
    (iii) SLE or polymyositis

Further reading

Simpson, J.A. (1974) *Disorders of Voluntary Muscle,* 3rd edn., ed. Walton, J.N. p. 653, Edinburgh: Churchill Livingstone

MYOTONIA

1. *Myotonia congenita*
    Thomson: Dominant
    Becker: Recessive, more severe and later onset
2. *Dystrophia myotonica*
    (i) Myotonia and muscle atrophy
    (ii) Characteristic facies with ptosis and frontal baldness
    (iii) Cataracts, gonadal atrophy, heart disease, hypoventilation, bone changes and dementia
3. *Paramyotonia congenita*
    Myotonia and weakness induced by cold, sometimes with fluctuation in serum potassium

Further reading

Walton, J.N. & Gardner-Medwin, D. (1974) *Disorders of Voluntary Muscle,* 3rd edn., ed. Walton, J.N. p. 592 Edinburgh: Churchill Livingstone.

CONGENITAL MYOPATHIES

   (i) Benign congenital hypotonia
  (ii) Central core disease
 (iii) Nemaline myopathy
 (iv) Myotubular myopathy
  (v) Congenital universal muscular hypoplasia
 (vi) Mitochondrial defects, e.g. megaconial myopathy
(vii) Arthrogryphosis multiplex congenita

METABOLIC AND ENDOCRINE MYOPATHIES

1. *Periodic paralysis*
   Se K may fall, rise or remain constant during attacks
2. *Glycogen storage diseases* (p. 116)
3. *Mitochondrial overactivity*
    (i) Hypermetabolic myopathy
   (ii) Malignant hyperpyrexia during anaesthesia
4. *Nutritional myopathy*
    (i) Kwashiorkor
   (ii) Vitamin E deficiency
5. *Drugs*
     (i) Alcohol (p. 93)
    (ii) Chloroquine
   (iii) Glucocorticoids, especially triamcinolone
    (iv) Vincristine
6. *Endocrine*
     (i) Hyper- or hypo-thyroidism
    (ii) Osteomalacia
   (iii) Acromegaly
    (iv) Cushing's syndrome
     (v) Hypoadrenalism
    (vi) Primary aldosteronism

Further reading

McArdle, B. (1974) *Disorders of Voluntary Muscle,* 3rd edn.,
ed. Walton, J.N. p. 721. Edinburgh: Churchill Livingstone

GLYCOGEN STORAGE DISEASES
TYPE I
Glucose - 6 - phosphatase deficiency (von Gierke) Hepatomegaly, retarded growth, hypoglycaemia, acidosis and ketonuria

TYPE II
1 - 4 Glucosidase deficiency (Pompe). Dyspnoea, cardiomegaly and weak hypotonic muscles.

TYPE III
Amylo - 1 - 6 - glucosidase deficiency (Cori). Clinically resembles Type I, but milder, with no hypoglycaemia.

TYPE IV
Amylo-transglucosidase deficiency (Anderson). Cirrhosis and death in early childhood. Very rare.

TYPE V
Muscle phosphorylase deficiency (McArdle). Pain, weakness and stiffness during exercise.

TYPE VI
(Her). Heterogeneous group with hepatomegaly and retarded growth.
Several other rare types exist.

Further reading
McArdle B. (1974) *Disorders of Voluntary Muscle,* 3rd edn., ed. Walton, J.N. p. 734. Edinburgh: Churchill Livingstone.

PROGRESSIVE MUSCULAR DYSTROPHIES
1. *X linked recessive ('Pseudo-hypertrophic')*
   (i) Duchenne (severe)
   (ii) Becker (milder and of later onset)
2. *Autosomal recessive*
   Limb girdle type (Erb)
3. *Autosomal dominant*
   (i) Facio-scapulo-humeral (Landouzy and Déjerine)
   (ii) Distal myopathy of late onset (Welander)
   (iii) Ocular myopathy (may also be either retinopathy or dysphagia)

Certain exceptions occur to this simple genetic classification

Further reading
Walton, J.N. & Gardner-Medwin, D. (1974) *Disorders of Voluntary Muscle,* 3rd edn., ed. Walton, J.N. p. 561 Edinburgh: Churchill Livingstone

FOUR SIMILAR SIGNS

1. *Kernig's sign.* To detect meningeal irritation

Straightening leg with hip flexed
produces pain and spasm of
hamstrings

2. *Brudzinski's sign.* To detect meningeal irritation

Flexing neck produces flexion of
lower limbs

3. *Thomas's test.* To detect fixed flexion deformity of the hip-joint

Eliminating lumbar lordosis
produces
flexion of the affected hip

4. *Straight-leg raising test.* To detect lesions of sciatic nerve or its
spinal roots

Straight-leg raising produces pain
below the normal full excursion

Endocrine and bone disease

DIABETES MELLITUS

Definition. Diabetes mellitus is a syndrome which merges with the normal, and diagnostic criteria are therefore arbitrary. The definition used by the British Diabetic Association depends on the oral glucose tolerance test, since more complex tests have failed to give better diagnostic discrimination. The test indicates diabetes if, after a 50g glucose load, the venous blood glucose concentration is 6.7 mmol/l (120mg/100 ml) or more at 2h., and 8.9 mmol/l (160mg/100 ml) or more at some other time during the test.

Further reading
Keen, H (1975) *Medicine,* 2nd series, **14,** 629.

Causes of diabetes mellitus
1. *Idiopathic*
    (i) Subclinical—Prediabetes (normal GTT, even after steroids
                                i.e. a retrospective diagnosis)
                    Latent (abnormal GTT after stress or steroids)
                    Asymptomatic (diabetic GTT)
    (ii) Clinical—'Juvenile onset'
                  'Maturity onset'
2. *Secondary to other disease*
    (i) Pancreatic disease (pancreatitis, Ca, haemochromatosis, etc)
    (ii) Cushing's syndrome
    (iii) Acromegaly
    (iv) Phaeochromocytoma
    (v) Cirrhosis
    (vi) Chronic renal failure
3. *Drugs*
    (i) Glucocorticoids
    (ii) Thiazides
    (iii) Oral contraceptives
    (iv) Diazoxide

Further reading
Hall, R. et al (1974) *Fundamentals of Clinical Endocrinology,* 2nd edn., p. 312. London: Pitman.

Chronic complications of diabetes mellitus
1. *Ocular*
    (i) Blurred vision due to fluctuations in blood sugar
    (ii) Cataracts
    (iii) Retinopathy:
        Venous engorgement
        Capillary microaneurysms
        'Blot' haemorrhages
        'Waxy' exudates
        Retinal infarcts ('cottonwool spots')
        Vitreous haemorrhage
        Retinitis proliferans
        Retinal detachment
    (vi) Rubeosis iridis (new blood vessels over iris)—may cause glaucoma
2. *Neurological*
    (i) Cerebral disturbance due to hyper- or hypoglycaemia
    (ii) Cerebral lesions due to atheroma
    (iii) Peripheral neuropathy
        a. Asymptomatic loss of ankle-jerks and vibration sense
        b. Painful subacute neuritis, usually in lower limbs
        c. Mononeuritis multiplex (often asymmetrical)
        d. Isolated cranial nerve lesions
        e. Autonomic neuropathy
    (iv) Diabetic pseudo-tabes
    (v) Diabetic amyotrophy
    (vi) 'Insulin neuritis' during stabilisation
3. *Renal*
    (i) Pyelonephritis, sometimes with papillary necrosis.
    (ii) Glomerulonephritis
        a. Kimmelstiel-Wilson (eosinophilic nodules in glomerular tuft)
        b. Proliferative, with sclerosed basement membrane
    (iii) Atherosclerosis and hypertensive vascular changes
4. *Vascular*
    Occlusion of large vessels (atheroma) or small vessels (endarteritis) may cause ischaemia of feet, myocardium, brain or kidneys
5. *Dermatological*
    (i) Fat atrophy or hypertrophy or fibrosis at insulin injection sites
    (ii) Ulcers due to neuropathy or ischaemia
    (iii) Infections, especially furuncles and Candidiasis
    (iv) Pigmented scars over shins ('diabetic dermopathy')
    (v) Xanthomata
    (vi) Necrobiosis lipoidica
    (vii) Widespread granuloma annulare
6. *Systemic infections*
    Incidence of TB, chronic urinary infections and deep mycoses is increased

Further reading
Keen, H. & Jarrett, J. (eds) (1975) *Complications of Diabetes.*
London: Arnold.

DIABETES AND PREGNANCY

Pregnancy produces a tendency to both keto-acidosis and fasting hypoglycaemia. This paradox is due to
1. Counteraction of maternal insulin by placental hormones
2. Removal of glucose by the fetus

COMPLICATIONS OF PREGNANCY IN THE DIABETIC

1. *Maternal morbidity*
    (i) Hydramnios
    (ii) Pre-eclampsia
    (iii) Pregnancy probably accelerates diabetic micro-angiopathy and some authors recommend abortion and sterilization in women with proliferative retinopathy or nephropathy
2. *Fetal mortality* Still-birth (5-10%) or neonatal death (5-10%) due to
    (i) Hyaline membrane disease (preterm delivery)
    (ii) Congenital anomalies (often cardiac or neurological)
3. *Fetal morbidity*
    (i) Macrosomia (excessive size)
    (ii) Hypoglycaemia
    (iii) Congenital anomalies
    (iv) Respiratory distress (due to pre-term delivery)
    (v) Hypocalcaemia (maternal hypercalcaemia suppresses the fetal parathyroid)

Further reading

Burrows, G.N. & Ferris, T.F. (1975) *Medical Complications during Pregnancy* p. 170. Philadelphia: Saunders
Essex, Nina. (1976) *British Journal of Hospital Medicine,* **15**, 333.

CAUSES OF HYPOGLYCAEMIA
1. *Starvation and exercise*
2. *Reaction to glucose ingestion*
   Functional
   Early diabetes mellitus
   Post-gastrectomy
3. *ß-cell overactivity*
   Insulinoma
   Hyperplasia
4. *Endocrine disease*
   Hypothyroidism
   Hypopituitarism
   Hypoadrenalism
5. *Drugs*
   Insulin
   Sulphonylureas
   Salicylates
   Paracetamol
   Ackee, etc.
6. *Sensitivity to:*
   Leucine
   Galactose, fructose
   Alcohol, tobacco
7. *Liver disease*
   Glycogen storage disease
   Hepatoma
8. *Neoplasm, esp. large fibrosarcoma*
9. *Idiopathic hypoglycaemia of infancy*
10. *Neonatal after fetal malnutrition*

Further reading

Marks, V. (1975) *Medicine,* 2nd series, **14,** 646.

CONGENITAL ADRENAL HYPERPLASIA

Cortisol, aldosterone and androgen synthesis may be affected depending on site of enzyme block.

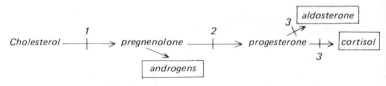

Site 1
Lipoid hyperplasia (C20 block)
Severe deficiency in all 3 hormones
Adrenal cortex filled with lipid

Site 2
3ß-hydroxysteroid dehydrogenase defect
Androgens unaffected

Site 3
21-hydroxylase defect
2 types
> (i) severe, with sodium loss in infancy
> (ii) mild, with virilism in female and pseudo-precocious puberty in male

Site 3
11ß-hydroxylase defect
Hypertension with virilisation
Rarer syndromes also exist

Further reading
Hall, R. et al (1974) *Fundamentals of Clinical Endocrinology* 2nd edn., p. 282. London: Pitman.

CAUSES OF ADRENAL INSUFFICIENCY

Primary
1. Acute or chronic gland destruction
     (i) Auto-immune adrenalitis
     (ii) Infection: TB , fungal, etc
     (iii) Infiltration: metastasis, amyloidosis, etc.
     (iv) Haemorrhage (especially Waterhouse-Friderichsen syndrome)
     (v) Surgery
2. Metabolic failure
     (i) Virilizing hyperplasia, e.g. C21-hydroxylase deficiency
     (ii) Enzyme inhibitors, e.g. metyrapone
     (iii) Cytotoxic drugs, e.g. opDDD

(contd.)

Secondary
1. Hypopituitarism
2. Suppression of hypothalamic-pituitary axis
    (i) Exogenous glucocorticoids
    (ii) Endogenous glucocorticoids, e.g. Cushing's syndrome
         following tumour removal

RENIN, ANGIOTENSIN AND ALDOSTERONE

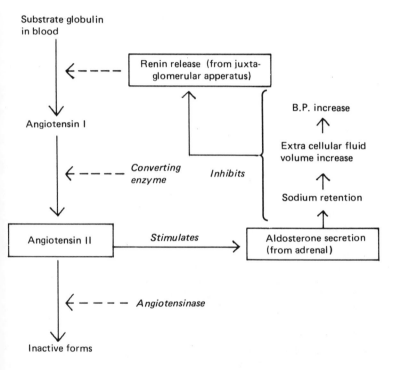

Saralasin competitively antagonises the acute pressor effect of angiotensin II

Further reading

Ledingham, J.G.G. (1975) *Medicine,* 2nd series, **29,** 1611
Brown, J.J. et al (1976) *Advanced Medicine, Symposium 12,* ed.
Peters, D.K., p. 407. London: Pitman

Hazards of systemic glucocorticoid therapy
1. Growth retardation in children
2. Cushingoid facies, buffalo hump
3. Adrenal suppression and atrophy
4. Weight gain, sodium and water retention, potassium depletion
5. Hypertension
6. Hyperglycaemia
7. Hyperlipidaemia
8. Infections, especially viral, TB and fungal
9. Osteoporosis, aseptic bone necrosis, ruptured Achilles tendon
10. Gastro-intestinal
    Dyspepsia
    Peptic ulcer and perforation
    Pancreatitis
11. CNS
    Euphoria
    Psychosis
    Increased intra-cranial pressure
    Increased tendency to epilepsy
12. Skin changes
    Thinning, striae and easy bruising
    Poor wound healing, enlargement of stasis ulcers or
    débridement injury
    Acne
    Hypertrichosis
13. Myopathy or muscle atrophy
14. Cataracts, and raised intra-ocular pressure
15. Amenorrhoea or premature menopause
16. Hypothermia
17. Withdrawal phenomena (vomiting, panniculitis, hypercalcaemia)
18. 'Rebound' of disease on reduction of dosage
19. Teratogenicity (fetal cleft palate)

Further reading

Myles, A.B. & Daly, J.R. (eds.) (1975) *Corticosteroid and ACTH Treatment.* London: Arnold.

CAUSES OF GYNAECOMASTIA
1. Hermaphroditism or pseudo-hermaphroditism (p. 128)
2. Endocrine
      Normal puberty and neonatal
      Hypothyroidism
      Thyrotoxicosis
      Hypoadrenalism
      Testicular atrophy
      Testicular and adrenal tumours
      Acromegaly
      Hypothalamic lesions
3. Cirrhosis
4. Carcinoma or lymphoma
5. Refeeding after malnutrition
6. Renal failure with dialysis
7. Paraplegia
8. Erythroderma
9. Leprosy
10. Drugs
      Sex hormones
      Spironolactone
      Amphetamine
      Reserpine
      Digitalis
      Methyldopa

CAUSES OF GALACTORRHOEA
1. Physiological (post-partum and neonatal)
2. Prolactin-secreting pituitary tumour
3. Pituitary stalk or hypothalamic lesion
4. Ectopic prolactin production e.g. bronchial Ca.
5. Drugs e.g.
      Phenothiazines
      Oral contraceptives
      Haloperidol
      Tricyclic antidepressants
      Methyldopa
      Meprobamate
      Reserpine
6. Chest wall injury (surgery, herpes zoster, mesothelioma)
      Probably stimulates neurological pathway of suckling reflex
7. Hysterectomy
8. Hypothyroidism

Further reading
Turkington, R.W. (1972) *Advances in Internal Medicine,* **18,** 363.

CAUSES OF AMENORRHOEA
Physiological
1. Pre-pubertal
2. Pregnancy
3. Menopausal

Pathological
1. *Anatomical*
    (i) Uterine anomaly
    (ii) Hysterectomy
    (iii) Cryptomenorrhoea
2. *Hypothalamic-pituitary axis*
    (i) 'Functional' amenorrhoea: change in environment, emotional upset, rapid change in weight
    (ii) Severe systemic disease: e.g. TB
    (iii) Hyperprolactinaemia
    (iv) Hypopituitarism
    (v) Thyrotoxicosis
    (vi) Drugs: oestrogen, progesterone, testosterone, glucocorticoids, spironolactone
3. *Primary ovarian disease*
    (i) Oophorectomy
    (ii) Irradiation
    (iii) Pelvic TB
4. *Virilizing syndromes*
    (i) Genetic intersex (p. 128)
    (ii) Ovarian
        Stein-Leventhal syndrome
        Virilizing tumours (p. 127)
    (iii) Adrenal
        Congenital adrenal hyperplasia
        Acquired virilizing adenoma or Ca.
5. *Oestrogen or progesterone excess*
    (i) Follicular or lutein retention cyst
    (ii) Sex cord stromal tumours

PROSTAGLANDINS
Possible physiological roles for prostaglandins
1. Feedback inhibition of neurotransmission
2. Luteolysis
3. Labour induction
4. Closure of ductus arteriosus
5. Renal autoregulation
6. Sperm transport
7. Ova transport

Further reading
Pike, J.E. (1976) *Journal of Investigative Dermatology,* **67,** 650
Bennett, A. (1973) *Advanced Medicine 9th Symposium,* ed. Walker, G., p. 182, London: Pitman.

OVARIAN TUMOURS

The multiplicity of terms used for ovarian tumours has led to confusion, and the W.H.O. Committee on Nomenclature (1973) has re-classified them into the following histological groups:

1. *Common 'epithelial' tumours*
   Probably originate from ovarian mesothelium
   e.g. serous
       mucinous
       endometrioid
       clear cell (mesonephroid), etc.
2. *Sex cord stromal tumours*
   e.g. granulosa—stromal cell
       androblastoma, from Sertoli or Leydig cells. These were formerly called arrhenoblastomata
3. *Lipoid cell tumours*
   Tumours (usually virilising), with an endocrine type architecture and large oval cells resembling lutein, Leydig or adrenocortical cells
   e.g. adrenal-like tumours
       luteomata
4. *Germ-cell tumours*
   Differentiate along embryonic lines
   e.g. dysgerminoma
       endodermal sinus (yolk sac)
       choriocarcinoma
       teratoma
5. *Gonadoblastoma*
   Almost invariably arise in abnormal gonads
6. *Soft tissue tumours not specific to ovary*
   e.g. vascular tumours
7. *Unclassified*
8. *Secondary (metastatic)*
   e.g. Krukenberg tumour
9. *Tumour-like conditions*

Most virilizing ovarian tumours are sex-cord or lipoid cell tumours

Further reading
Fox, H. & Langley, F.A. (1976) *Tumours of the Ovary*. London: Heinemann.

CAUSES OF PRECOCIOUS PUBERTY

A. True precocity (premature activation of pituitary—hypothalamic axis)
  1. *Constitutional* (usually female, may be familial)
  2. *Secondary*
      (i) Tumours near the hypothalamus, e.g. pinealoma, hamartoma, teratoma etc.
      (ii) Brain damage, e.g. encephalitis, hydrocephalus, etc.
      (iii) Polyostotic fibrous dysplasia (Albright's syndrome)
      (iv) Hepatic cell carcinoma

B. Pseudo-precocity (secondary sexual development with immature gonads)
Overproduction of androgen or oestrogen by
      (i) Disease of ovary, testis or adrenal
      (ii) Teratoma
      (iii) Exogenous hormone

Further reading

Hall, R. et al (1974) in *Fundamentals of Clinical Endocrinology* 2nd edn., p. 262. London: Pitman.

INTERSEXUAL STATES

True hermaphrodites have both testicular and ovarian elements in the gonads
Male pseudo-hermaphrodites have testes but are feminized
Female pseudo-hermaphrodites have ovaries but are virilised

Causes
  1. *Genetic*
      (i) Turner's: XO
      (ii) Chromatin positive ovarian dysgenesis
            Abnormal X
            Mosaics
      (iii) Klinefelter's: XXY
      (vi) 'Super-females': XXX, etc.
      (v) 'Super-males': XYY, etc.
      (vi) Mosaics: XY/XO, XX/XY, etc.
      (vii) Gonadal dysgenesis: female phenotype
  2. *Hormonal*
Female
      (i) Congenital adrenal hyperplasia
      (ii) Virilising tumour of mother during pregnancy
      (iii) Sex hormones given to mother during pregnancy, e.g. to prevent abortion
Male
            End-organ unresponsiveness to androgens

THE THYROID
CAUSES OF HYPOTHYROIDISM

A. Primary (thyroid gland failure)
1. Congenital
   (i) Absence or maldevelopment of thyroid gland
   (ii) Endemic cretinism (maternal iodine deficiency)
   (iii) Dyshormonogenesis (enzyme defects affecting hormone synthesis)
      e.g. peroxidase deficiency
2. Auto-immune thyroiditis
3. Iatrogenic
   (i) Surgery
   (ii) Irradiation
   (iii) Anti-thyroid drugs
4. Dietary iodine deficiency
5. Acquired enzyme defects due to goitrogens (dietary or drugs)
6. Riedel's thyroiditis (very rare)

B. Secondary (TSH deficiency)
1. Hypopituitarism
2. Rarely hypothalamic lesion (TRH deficiency)

CAUSES OF HYPERTHYROIDISM
1. Graves' disease and toxic multinodular goitre
2. Toxic adenoma
3. Iatrogenic
   (i) Overdosage with thyroid hormone
   (ii) Following administration of iodine to goitrous patient (Jod-Basedow phenomenon)
4. Ectopic TSH secretion by neoplasm e.g. choriocarcinoma
5. Ectopic thyroid secretion by struma ovarii

Further reading

Hall, R. et al (1974) *Fundamentals of Clinical Endocrinology* 2nd edn., p. 68. London: Pitman.

TESTS OF THYROID FUNCTION

1. **Measurement of circulating thyroid hormones**
    (i) Thyroxine (T_4)
        Affected by level of thyroid hormone-binding globulin (TBG)
        Does not detect T_3 thyrotoxicosis (e.g. in iodine deficiency)
    (ii) Tri-iodothyronine (T_3)
        Detects T_3 thyrotoxicosis
    (iii) T_3 resin-uptake
        Determined by the degree of saturation of TBG with thyroid hormone

    (iv) Protein-bound iodine (PBI)
    (v) 'Free thyroxine index'
        The product of PBI and T_3 resin uptake. It is independent of the level of TBG
    (vi) Thyrotrophin (TSH)
        Increased in primary hypothyroidism
2. **Radio-iodine uptake tests, (I^{131}, I^{125}, Tc)**
3. **Peripheral tissue response tests**
    Useful in diagnosis of hypothyroidism only
    (i) Tendon reflex duration
    (ii) Se cholesterol
    (iii) ECG
    (iv) Clinical response to thyroxine

4. T₃ suppresssion test
Suppression of I¹³¹ uptake by T_3 is strong evidence against hyperthyroidism. Useful in distinguishing high I¹³¹ uptake of iodine deficiency from hyperthyroidism

5. TRH Test
The TSH response following intra-venous TRH is now replacing the T_3 suppression test for the diagnosis of thyroid autonomy.
Hypothyroidism → an exaggerated rise of an already increased TSH.
Hyperthyroidism → no response of a depressed TSH. Useful for diagnosis of doubtful hyperthyroidism and ophthalmic Graves' disease

6. TSH Stimulation test
TSH stimulates I¹³¹ uptake in secondary, but not in primary, hypothyroidism

7. Perchlorate discharge test
Detects inability of thyroid to bind iodine (the commonest type of dyshormonogenesis)

Further reading

Hall, R. et al (1974) *Fundamentals of Clinical Endocrinology* 2nd edn., pp. 75 & 453. London: Pitman.
Havard, C.W.H. (1975) *British Journal of Hospital Medicine,* **14,** 239.

THYROID HORMONE BINDING GLOBULIN (TBG)
Causes of increased TBG
   1. Pregnancy
   2. Oestrogen therapy
   3. Clofibrate

Causes of decreased TBG
   1. Hypoproteinaemia (e.g. nephrotic syndrome)
   2. Acromegaly
   3. Glucocorticoids, androgens and anabolic steroids

Causes of reduced TBG binding
   1. Renal failure
   2. Salicylates, phenytoin, phenylbutazone

Further reading

Havard, C.W.H. (1975) *British Journal of Hospital Medicine,* **14,** 239.

HYPOTHALAMIC REGULATORY HORMONES

Thyrotrophin releasing hormone—TRH
Releases
- (i) TSH and prolactin in both sexes
- (ii) FSH in men
- (iii) GH in some patients with acromegaly and renal failure

Luteinising/Follicle-stimulating hormone releasing factor— LH/FSH-RH
Releases
- (i) LH and FSH in both sexes
- (ii) GH in some patients with acromegaly

Somatostatin—GH-RIH
Suppresses
- (i) GH in normal subjects and acromegalic patients
- (ii) TSH response to TRH
- (iii) TSH secretion in hypothyroidism
- (iv) ACTH secretion in Nelson's syndrome (post-adrenalectomy)
- (v) Insulin, glucagon and gastrin release

Conditions associated with an impaired TSH response to TRH
1. Thyroid disease
   - (i) Hyperthyroidism
   - (ii) Pre-hyperthyroidism
   - (iii) Euthyroid patients being treated for hyperthyroidism
   - (iv) Ophthalmic Graves' disease
   - (v) Multinodular goitre
2. Hypothalamic disease
3. Acromegaly or hypopituitarism
4. Cushing's disease
5. Depression
6. Starvation
7. Drugs—glucocorticoids, thyroid hormones, L-dopa
8. Some normal people

Further reading

Hall, R. & Gomez-Pan, A. (1975) *Advanced Medicine Symposium 11,* ed. Lant, A.F., p. 234. London: Pitman.

METABOLIC BONE DISEASE
Causes of osteomalacia and rickets
1. *Deficiency of cholecalciferol (vit. D)*
    (i) Prematurity, multiple pregnancy, prolonged breast feeding and lack of UV predispose to rickets
    (ii) Dietary
    (iii) Post-gastrectomy (probably dietary)
    (iv) Malabsorption (p. 42)
    (v) Anticonvulsants (liver enzyme induction)
2. *Renal causes*
    (i) Chronic renal failure
    (ii) Idiopathic hypercalciuria
    (iii) Fanconi syndrome (p. 146)
    (iv) Tubular acidosis
3. *Hepatic disease (disturbed vit. D. metabolism)*
4. *Hypo-phosphatasia*

Causes of osteoporosis
1. Senile osteoporosis
2. Immobilisation
3. Endocrine
      Sex hormone deficiency e.g. premature menopause
      Cushing's or glucocorticoid therapy
      Hyperthyroidism
      Diabetes mellitus
4. Deficiency of oestrogen, androgen, protein, vit. C or calcium
5. Chronic renal failure
6. Miscellaneous
      Alcoholism
      Osteogenesis imperfecta
      Werner Rothmund syndrome
      Glycogen storage disease
      Cirrhosis in children
      Systemic mastocytosis or heparin infusion
      Homocystinuria
7. Localized osteoporosis, e.g. rheumatoid arthritis
8. Idiopathic osteoporosis of young people

Further reading
Nordin, B.E.C. (1973) *Metabolic Bone and Stone Disease.* p. 1.
Edinburgh: Churchill Livingstone

Causes of hypocalcaemia
1. Hypoparathyroidism
   (i) Post-thyroidectomy
   (ii) Idiopathic (sometimes with hypoadrenalism and Candidiasis)
2. Deficiency of cholecalciferol (p. 133)
3. Malabsorption
4. Chronic renal failure or Fanconi syndrome (p. 146)
5. Hypoalbuminaemia
6. Neonatal hypocalcaemia
   (i) High-phosphate artificial feeds
   (ii) Associated with low birth-weight and hypoglycaemia
   (iii) Parathyroid suppression due to maternal hyperparathyroidism
7. Acute pancreatitis
8. Pseudo-hypoparathyroidism

Causes of hypercalcaemia
1. Hyperparathyroidism
2. Malignancy with or without metastases
3. Myelomatosis, (rarely lymphoma or leukaemia)
4. Vit. D sensitivity, especially sarcoidosis
5. Vit. D excess
6. Milk-alkali syndrome
7. Infantile hypercalcaemia
8. Thyrotoxicosis
9. Hypothyroidism, especially in infants
10. Steroid withdrawal (iatrogenic, or acute hypoadrenalism)
11. Paget's disease (when immobilised)
12. Immobilisation (very rarely)

Further reading
Watson, L. (1975) *Medicine,* 2nd series, **8,** 341.

	Se Calcium	Se Phosphate	Parathormone Infusion
Hypoparathyroidism	Low	High	Marked response
Pseudo-hypopara-thyroidism	Low	High	No response
Pseudo-pseudo-hypoparathyroidism	Normal	Normal	No response

Causes of hypercalciuria
1. All causes of hypercalcaemia, if renal function is normal
2. Renal tubular acidosis
3. Progressive osteoporosis
4. Cushing's syndrome
5. Acromegaly
6. Prolonged immobilisation
7. Excess dietary calcium
8. Idiopathic hypercalciuria

Further reading

Smith, L.H. & Williams, H.E. (1971) *Diseases of the Kidney,* 2nd edn., ed. Strauss, M.B. & Welt, L.G., p. 981. Boston: Little Brown

Tests to distinguish hyperparathyroidism from other causes of hypercalcaemia
1. *Steroid suppression test*
   Hypercalcaemia due to hyperparathyroidism is not suppressed by cortisol 40 mg. tds.
2. *Plasma phosphate*
   Consistently low PO_4 suggests primary hyperparathyroidism
3. *Phosphate excretion tests* (e.g. PEI, p. 197)
   Based on blockage of net phosphate reabsorption by parathormone
4. *Acid-base status*
   Patients with hyperparathyroidism have hyperchloraemic acidosis
   Other hypercalcaemic patients have hypochloraemic alkalosis
5. *Parathormone radioimmunoassay*
6. *Plasma alkaline phosphatase*
   Increased in patients with X-ray signs of hyperparathyroidism (osteoblastic activity)
7. *Calcium tolerance tests* (urinary phosphate excretion after calcium infusion)
   Parathormone production is not suppressed in hyperparathyroidism. Of limited value due to false positives and negatives

Causes of soft-tissue calcification
1. *Dystrophic*
Occurs in abnormal tissue, often with impaired blood supply.
    (i) Inflammatory foci e.g. TB
    (ii) Neoplasia and naevi
    (iii) Parasites e.g. cysticercosis
    (iv) Haematoma
    (v) Gravitational oedema (esp. leg ulcers)
    (vi) Systemic sclerosis, dermatomyositis
    (vii) Ehlers-Danlos syndrome (cutis hyperelastica)
2. *Metastatic (metabolic)*
Calcification of normal tissue, e.g. kidneys or arteries, due to a metabolic abnormality such as hypercalcaemia or hypervitaminosis D. Intra-cranial calcification occurs in hypoparathyroidism and pseudo-hypoparathyroidism
3. *Secondary to bone or joint disease*
e.g. calcified cartilage, tendon or periosteum
4. *Idiopathic calcification*
    (i) Calcinosis circumscripta
    (ii) Calcinosis universalis
    (iii) Myositis ossificans

Further reading
Nordin, B.E.C. (1973) *Metabolic Bone and Stone Disease*, p. 244. Edinburgh: Churchill Livingstone.

Causes of discrete translucencies in a skull X-ray
1. Hyperparathyroidism
2. Myelomatosis
3. Metastatic deposits, esp. neuroblastoma
4. Leukaemia
5. Sickle-cell anaemia
6. Histiocytosis X, esp. Hand-Schuller-Christian disease
7. Sarcoidosis
8. Congenital cranial lacunae

Causes of bilateral frontal 'bossing'
1. Paget's
2. Rickets
3. Achondroplasia
4. Congenital hydrocephalus
5. Basal cell naevi syndrome (Gorlin's)

Causes of 'bowing' of tibia
1. Paget's
2. Rickets
3. Syphilis or yaws
4. Polyostotic fibrous dysplasia (Albright's)

MULTIPLE ENDOCRINE ADENOMATOSIS SYNDROMES

Type I. Werner's syndrome
Tumours of parathyroid, pituitary and pancreas

Parathyroid Adenoma or hyperplasia in 90%

Pituitary Adenoma in 65% (usually nonfunctional)

Pancreas
- (i) Islet-cell tumours with peptic ulceration (Zollinger-Ellison)
- (ii) Insulinoma
- (iii) Glucagonoma, with necrolytic migratory erythema, stomatitis, weight loss and diabetes
- (iv) Delta-cell hyperplasia with watery diarrhoea, hypokolaemia and fasting achlorhydria (Werner-Morrison)

Other reported lesions include adrenal hyperplasia or tumour, various thyroid lesions, carcinoid, schwannoma and thymoma

Type II. Sipple's syndrome
Tumours of thyroid, adrenal medulla and occasionally parathyroid adenoma or hyperplasia

Thyroid Medullary carcinoma which may secrete calcitonin, ACTH, serotonin or prostaglandin

Adrenal Phaeochromocytoma' which may be asymptomatic. Some patients also have the 'mucosal neuroma' syndrome with pigmentation, thick lips, tongue or eyelid neuromas, lax joints and a Marfanoid body habitus

Further reading
Schimke, R.N. (1976) *Advances in Internal Medicine,* **21,** 249.

Conditions associated with familial phaeochromocytoma
1. Multiple endocrine adenomatosis, Type II
2. Neurofibromatosis (von Recklinghausen)
3. Cerebellar haemangioblastoma(von Hippel-Lindau)
4. Basal-cell naevi syndrome (Gorlin)

Renal disease

CAUSES OF CHRONIC RENAL FAILURE

1. *Glomerulonephritis*
   (i) Immune-complex nephritis
       Primary e.g. post-Streptococcal
       Secondary e.g. Henoch-Schönlein vasculitis
   (ii) Anti-glomerular basement membrane nephritis
       e.g. Goodpasture's nephritis with pulmonary bleeding
2. *Infections*
   Chronic pyelonephritis
   Renal TB (now uncommon)
3. *Obstruction*
   Stone, stricture, stenosis, etc.
4. *Incomplete recovery from acute renal failure* (esp. cortical necrosis)
5. *Vascular*
   Ischaemia
   Hypertension
6. *'Collagen vascular' diseases*
   Systemic vasculitis (PN etc, p. 159)
   SLE
   Systemic sclerosis
   'Haemolytic uraemic' syndrome
   Thrombotic thrombocytopenia of Moschcowitz
7. *Metabolic*
   Diabetes mellitus
   Amyloidosis
   Gout
   Hypercalcaemia (p. 134)
   Chronic hypokalaemia
   Drugs (esp. analgesic abuse) and toxins (e.g. heavy metals)
   Dysproteinaemia (esp. myelomatosis)
8. *Primary tubular disease*
   Fanconi syndrome (p. 146)
   Tubular acidosis
9. *Congenital anomalies*
   Polycystic kidney
   Renal hypoplasia
10. *Miscellaneous rare diseases*
    e.g. Radiation nephritis
       Balkan nephropathy
       Angiokeratoma corporis diffusum (Fabry's disease)
       Alport's disease (familial nephritis with deafness)

DIALYSIS
Possible indications for short-term dialysis
1. Acute renal failure
    (i) Hyperkalaemia > 7 mmol/l
    (ii) Arterial pH < 7.15
    (iii) Blood urea > 35 mmol/l
    (iv) Rapidly rising blood urea
2. Fluid overload
3. Uncontrolled hypercalcaemia
4. Gross electrolyte disturbance
5. Poisoning with salicylates
            barbiturates
            ethanol
6. Acute-on-chronic renal failure prior to establishing conservative therapy

Possible indications for long-term haemodialysis
1. Failure of conservative management
2. Se. creatinine > 1200 μmols/l
3. GFR < 3 ml/min
4. Progression of bone disease
5. Progression of neuropathy
6. Onset of pericarditis (peritoneal dialysis may be necessary initially to avoid haemopericarditis)

Neurological complications of renal failure
1. Encephalopathy with dementia
2. Epilepsy
3. Psychoses, esp. depression
4. Amaurosis
5. Cerebro-vascular accident
6. Basal ganglia lesions (tremor, rigidity, etc.)
7. Cranial neuropathy
8. Central pontine myelopathy
9. Peripheral neuropathy
10. Myopathy or muscle cramps
11. 'Restless leg' syndrome
12. Complications of therapy, e.g. viral or fungal CNS infection due to immunosuppressives
13. Lymphoma of CNS following renal transplant

Further reading
Neary, D. (1976) *British Journal of Hospital Medicine,* **15,** 122.

Renal causes of polycythaemia
-1. Hypernephroma
-2. Polycystic disease
- 3. Hydronephrosis
4. Renal artery stenosis
5. Transplantation

GLOMERULONEPHRITIS

Histological classification
1. *Minimal lesion* (no change on light microscopy)
2. *Membranous* (no cellular proliferation)
3. *Proliferative glomerulonephritis (PGN)*
   Each of the 3 cellular elements, epithelial, endothelial or
   mesangial, may show proliferative changes together or singly.
   (i) Active diffuse endothelial PGN
   (ii) Mesangial PGN
   (iii) Rapidly progressive PGN with extensive epithelial
         crescents
   (iv) Mesangiocapillary PGN
   (v) Focal PGN (affects only some parts of some glomeruli)
   (vi) Chronic endothelial PGN
4. *Focal glomerulosclerosis*
5. *Advanced sclerosing lesions*

   3(i) and 3(ii) are commonly post-streptococcal

Clinical syndromes of glomerulonephritis
1. Acute nephritis
2. Nephrotic syndrome
3. Persistent proteinuria
4. Recurrent haematuria or loin pain
5. Chronic renal failure
6. Acute oliguric renal failure (rare)

Antigens implicated in glomerulonephritis
1. *Bacterial*
   Streptococcal (β haemolytic, type 12)
   Staphylococci (in bact. endocarditis and in 'shunt' nephritis)
   Mycobact. leprae
   Treponema pallidum
   Salmonella typhi
2. *Viral*
   Australia antigen, varicella, mumps, EB virus, Coxsackie B
3. *Protozoal*
   Plasmodium malariae, schistosoma, toxoplasma
4. *Others*
   DNA (in SLE)
   Thyroglobulin (in auto-immune thyroiditis)
   Cryoglobulin
   Tumour antigens
   Carcino-embryonic antigen (in Ca colon)
   Drugs, e.g. penicillamine, heroin

Further reading

Cameron, J.S. (1972) *Renal Disease* 3rd edn., ed. Sir Douglas Black, p. 295. Oxford: Blackwell.
Sissons, J.G.P. (1975) *Medicine,* 2nd series, **6,**256.

CAUSES OF NEPHROTIC SYNDROME

1. *Glomerulonephritis (p. 140)*
   Accounts for 80% of cases
2. *Metabolic*
   - (i) Diabetes mellitus ⌐
   - (ii) Amyloidosis
   - (iii) Lymphoma
   - (iv) Extra-renal malignancy
   - (v) Dysproteinaemia, esp. myelomatosis
   - (vi) Dermatoses
   - (vii) Sickle cell anaemia
   - (viii) Myxoedema
3. *'Collagen vascular' disease*
   esp. SLE and vasculitis
4. *Infection*
   - (i) Malaria
   - (ii) Cytomegalic inclusion disease
   - (iii) Syphilis
   - (iv) Bacterial endocarditis
   - (v) Staphylococcal septicaemia
   - (vi) Leprosy
5. *Mechanical*
   Renal artery stenosis
   Renal vein thrombosis (may be cause or effect)
   Inf. vena caval thrombosis
   Constrictive pericarditis
   Renal carcinoma
   Chyluria
6. *Drugs*
   Mercurials, troxidone, penicillamine, etc.
7. *Hypersensitivity*
   - (i) Se sickness, bee stings, poison ivy, pollen, etc.
   - (ii) Smallpox vaccination
8. *Congenital and familial*

Further reading

Robson, J.S. (1972) *Renal Disease*. 3rd edn., ed. Sir Douglas Black.
p. 331. Oxford: Blackwell.

Causes of renal vein thrombosis

1. Nephrotic syndrome of any cause
2. Renal amyloid
3. Hypernephroma
4. Trauma, including cannulation
5. Dehydration, especially in infancy

Causes of papillary necrosis
1. Analgesic abuse, esp. phenacetin
2. Obstructive uropathy, esp. with infection
3. Acute pyelonephritis, esp. in diabetes mellitus
4. Sickle cell disease
5. Renal T.B.
6. Dysproteinaemia

Chronic interstitial nephritis
Defined as renal disease with the histological features of chronic pyelonephritis but with no evidence of bacterial infection. Many renal diseases produce interstitial changes, including:
1. Obstruction
2. Nephrocalcinosis
3. Potassium depletion
4. Hyperuricaemia
5. Analgesic abuse
6. Acute tubular necrosis
7. Irradiation
8. Lead poisoning
9. Balkan nephropathy

Further reading

Freedman, L.R. (1971) *Diseases of the Kidney,* 2nd edn., p. 667, ed. Strauss, M.B. & Welt, L.G. Boston: Little Brown.

Causes of 'sterile' pyuria
1. Renal TB
2. Analgesic nephropathy
3. Renal calculi
4. Urinary infection treated with chemotherapy
5. Drugs
    (i) Analgesics
    (ii) Diuretics
    (iii) Iron sorbitol citric acid complex (Jectofer)
6. Non-specific urethritis

NEPHROCALCINOSIS AND RENAL STONES
Causes of renal stones
1. *Calcium stones* (oxalate, phosphate, mixed magnesium-ammonium, etc.)
   - (i) With hypercalcaemia
     - Primary hyperparathyroidism
     - Sarcoidosis
     - Idiopathic hypercalcaemia of infancy
     - Chronic milk-alkali syndrome
     - Vit. D excess
   - (ii) With normocalcaemia
     - Idiopathic hypercalciuria
     - Prolonged bed rest
     - Primary renal tubular acidosis
     - Urinary tract infection
     - Hyperoxaluria
     - Medullary sponge kidney
2. *Uric acid stones*
   - (i) With hyperuricaemia
     - Gout
     - Polycythaemia, leukaemia, malignancy, etc.
     - Chronic metabolic acidosis, e.g. glycogen storage disease
     - Lesch-Nyhan syndrome
   - (ii) With normouricaemia
     - Idiopathic
     - Acid, concentrated urine (e.g. desert climates)
3. *Cystine stones*
   - (i) Congenital cystinuria
   - (ii) Hereditary cystinosis

RADIO-OPAQUE STONES	NON-OPAQUE STONES
Calcium	Uric acid
Mg-ammonium phosphate	Xanthine
Cystine	Matrix
Silicate	

Differential diagnosis
Blood clot
Sloughed papillae
Tumour
Varices

Radiographic nephrocalcinosis
1. *Coarse, medullary*

Causes
   (i) Primary hyperparathyroidism
  (ii) Primary renal tubular acidosis
 (iii) Sarcoidosis
 (iv) Milk-alkali syndrome
  (v) Primary hyperoxaluria (oxalosis)
 (vi) Idiopathic hypercalciuria
(vii) Idiopathic

2. *Localised*

Causes
   (i) Medullary sponge kidney
     (calcified collecting ducts)
  (ii) Renal neoplasm
 (iii) Cyst or haematoma
 (iv) Papillary necrosis
  (v) TB
 (vi) Hydatid cyst

3. *Diffuse, cortical (Rare)*

Causes
  (i) Chronic glomerulonephritis
 (ii) Old cortical necrosis

Further reading
Wrong, O.M. & Feest, T.G. (1976) *Advanced Medicine, Symposium 12*. ed. Peters, D.K. p. 394 London: Pitman.

Execretion urography in acute renal failure
Now regarded as safe, providing dehydration is avoided (especial
care needed in patients with liver failure, diabetes and
myelomatosis)
The evolution of the nephrogram is helpful—

Type 1. Immediate, faint, persisting
Chronic glomerulo-nephritis

Type 2. Increasingly dense with time
Obstruction
Hypotension or ischaemia
Severe glomerulonephritis

Type 3. Immediate, dense, persisting
Acute tubular necrosis
Oliguric pyelonephritis

Type 4. No nephrogram
Anuric glomerulonephritis
Renal infarction
Severe interstitial nephritis
In obstructive uropathy there may also be asymmetry of renal size,
and a slowly developing dense pyelogram

Further reading

Cattell, W.R. (1975) *Recent advances in renal disease*, ed. Jones,
N.F. No. 1, p. 21. Edinburgh: Churchill Livingstone
Fry, I.K. (1975) *Medicine,* 2nd series, **29,** 1618.

Causes of small kidneys
1. Chronic glomerulonephritis (smooth outline)
2. Chronic pyelonephritis (irregular outline)
3. Other chronic nephropathy, e.g. interstitial nephritis
4. Renal artery stenosis
5. Atrophy following obstruction
6. Congenital renal hypoplasia (prone to infection)

Causes of large kidney (or kidneys)
1. Polycystic disease
2. Hydronephrosis
3. Hypernephroma
4. Hypertrophy following contra-lateral nephrectomy or failure
5. Nephrotic syndrome
6. Acute pyelonephritis
7. Compulsive water, beer and cider drinker
Also consider the possibility of peri-renal haematoma

RENAL TUBULAR DISORDERS

Single transport defects

1. *Impaired reabsorption*
   Water—nephrogenic diabetes insipidus
   Na or K—distal tubular damage e.g. chronic pyelonephritis
   Calcium—idiopathic hypercalciuria
   Phosphate—vitamin D resistant rickets
   Glucose—renal glycosuria
   Amino acids—see p. 147
   Xanthine—xanthinuria
2. *Excessive reabsorption*
   Phosphate—pseudo-hypoparathyroidism

Multiple transport defects

1. *Impaired acidification*
   (i) Renal tubular acidosis
   (ii) Chronic pyelonephritis
   (iii) Hypokalaemia
   (iv) Hypercalcaemia
   (v) Hydronephrosis
2. *Impaired reabsorption and acidification*
   (Fanconi syndrome) e.g.
   (i) Hereditary cystinosis (Lignac-Fanconi)
   (ii) Toxins—cadmium, Hg, lead
   (iii) Drugs—neomycin, outdated tetracycline
   (iv) Galactosaemia
   (v) Hepatolenticular degeneration
   (vi) Nephrotic syndrome
   (vii) Lowe's oculo-cerebro-renal syndrome

Further reading

Gabriel, R. (1974) *Postgraduate Nephrology,* p. 142 London:
Butterworth.

AMINO-ACIDURIA

Four groups with separate transport systems
1. Proline, hydroxyproline and glycine
2. Dibasic: cystine, ornithine, arginine and lysine (COAL)
3. Dicarboxylic: glutamic and aspartic acids
4. Monoamino-monocarboxylic: all the rest

Causes of aminoaciduria
1. *Pure 'overflow'* due to raised plasma levels
   Amino-acid infusion
   Liver failure
   Phenylketonuria
   Maple-syrup urine
   Histidinaemia
   Glycinaemia
2. *A specific transport defect*
   Cystinuria
   Hartnup disease (malabsorption, ataxia and pellagrous rash)
3. *Generalised proximal tubular damage* (Fanconi syndrome, p. 146)
4. *Mixed 'overflow' and renal*
   Citrullinuria
   Prolinaemia

SOME CAUSES OF 'DARK COLOURED' URINE
1. Concentration
2. Bile
3. Blood, haemoglobinuria or myoglobinuria
4. Methaemoglobinuria
5. Porphyria
6. Alkaptonuria
7. Melaninuria
8. Beetroot, dyes in sweets, etc.

DRUG-INDUCED RENAL DISEASE

1. **Acute renal failure** (20% of cases are due to drugs)
    Over 70 drugs implicated, and a variety of mechanisms,
    - (i) Direct toxicity (dose-related)
      e.g. cephaloridine, amphotericin B
    - (ii) Hypersensitivity
      e.g. penicillin, sulphonamides
    - (iii) Obstruction due to crystal formation
      e.g. sulphonamides
    - (iv) 'Osmotic nephrosis'
      e.g. low MW dextran infusion

    Tetracyclines cause two distinct disorders—
    - a. Renal failure (due to increased urea production, increased sodium excretion and reduced urine-concentrating ability)
    - b. Degraded tetracyclines cause proximal tubular defects (Fanconi syndrome)

2. **Drug-induced LE**
    (especially in slow acetylators), (p. 178)
3. **Nephrotic syndrome** (p. 141)
4. **Papillary necrosis**
    Analgesics, especially phenacetin
5. **Retro-peritoneal fibrosis**
    e.g. methysergide, ergotamine, methyldopa
6. **Metabolic effects**
    - (i) Increased protein breakdown, e.g. glucocorticoids
    - (ii) Electrolyte disturbance, e.g. drugs causing diarrhoea
    - (iii) Nephrocalcinosis, e.g. vitamin D overdosage
    - (iv) Renal calculi, e.g. 'milk-alkali' syndrome
    - (v) Urate nephropathy, e.g. cytotoxins for malignancy
    - (vi) Impaired urine-concentrating ability, e.g. demethylchlortetracycline, lithium
    - (vii) Inappropriate ADH secretion (p. 152)
7. **Neoplasm**
    Renal pelvis mesothelial tumour, e.g analgesics

Further reading
Curtis, J.R. (1977) *British Medical Journal* **2**, 242, and 375.

ACID-BASE BALANCE

These headings reflect changes in extra-cellular fluid only, e.g. in metabolic alkalosis there is an associated intra-cellular acidosis

1. RESPIRATORY ACIDOSIS (Low pH, High CO_2 content)
    Any cause of hypoventilation (p. 23)

2. RESPIRATORY ALKALOSIS (High pH, Low CO_2 content)
    Any cause of hyperventilation (p. 23)

3. METABOLIC ACIDOSIS (Low pH, Low CO_2 content)

    Causes
    (i) *Ingestion of hydrion or 'potential acid'*
       Diets high in protein and fat
       Ammonium chloride, salicylates, calcium chloride, etc.
       'Dilution acidaemia' due to rapid saline infusion
    (ii) *Metabolic overproduction of hydrions*
       Hypercatabolic states
       Ketosis, e.g. starvation, diabetes mellitus
       Lactic acidosis (p. 150)
    (iii) *Intestinal loss of base*
       Diarrhoea
       Fistulae
    (iv) *Renal causes*
       a. Acute or chronic failure
       b. Defective hydrion secretion
          Renal tubular acidosis
          Pyelonephritis
          Hydronephrosis
       c. Extra-renal causes
          Carbonic anhydrase inhibitors
          Addison's disease
          Uretero-sigmoidostomy

4. METABOLIC ALKALOSIS (High pH, High CO_2 content)
    Causes
    Ingestion of alkali, e.g. $NaHCO_3$
    Vomiting, or gastric aspiration
    Hypokalaemia (p. 150)

5. MIXED DISORDERS
    e.g. Respiratory and metabolic acidosis in hypoventilated hypoxic patients
       Respiratory alkalosis and metabolic acidosis in salicylate poisoning

Causes of lactic acidosis
1. *Poor tissue perfusion or hypoxia,* e.g. 'shock'
2. *Metabolic disease*
   Renal failure
   Hepatic failure
   Infection
   Diabetes mellitus
3. *Drugs*
   Phenformin or metformin
   Ethanol or methanol
   Fructose, etc.
4. *Ingestion of 'lactic acid' milk*
5. *Congenital*
   G6P deficiency, etc.

N.B. An increased anion gap ($[Na^+] + [K^+]$) − ($[Cl^-] + [HCO_3^-]$) is helpful in diagnosis if blood lactate estimation cannot be performed.

Further reading
Woods, H.F. (1974) *Advanced Medicine, Symposium 10,* ed.
Ledingham, J.G.G. p. 53 London: Pitman.
Alberti, K.G.M.M. & Natress, M. (1977) *Lancet,* **2,** 25

Causes of hypokalaemia
1. *Increased renal loss*
   (i) Diuresis
       Drugs
       Diabetes mellitus
   (ii) Mineralocorticoid excess
       Primary aldosteronism (Conn's tumour)
       Cushing's
       Ingestion of liquorice or carbenexolone
   (iii) Primary renal disease
       Diuretic phase of acute renal failure
       Chronic pyelonephritis
       Fanconi syndrome (p. 146)
       Renal tubular acidosis
       Renal ischaemia
2. *Increased intestinal loss*
   Diarrhoea
   Vomiting
   Aspiration
   Fistulae
   Resonium A
3. *Decreased intake*
   Dietary lack
   Malabsorption
4. *Familial periodic paralysis*
5. *I.V. insulin*

Further reading
Wilkinson, R. (1975) *Medicine,* 2nd series, **7,** 334.

Causes of hypernatraemia
1. *Inadequate water intake*
   Lack of water, inability to drink, etc.
2. *Inadequate water retention*
   Diabetes insipidus
3. *Excessive sodium intake*
   Diet or drugs (oral or intravenous)
4. *Excessive sodium retention*
   Hyperaldosteronism

Causes of hyponatraemia
1. *Excessive water intake*
   Oral (polydipsia) or intravenous
2. *Excessive water retention*
   Inappropriate ADH secretion
3. *Inadequate sodium intake* (rare)
4. *Inadequate sodium retention*
      (i) Vomiting, diarrhoea
     (ii) Hypoadrenalism
    (iii) 'Salt-losing nephritis'

CAUSES OF JAUNDICE WITH URAEMIA
1. Infections
      (i) Gram-negative septicaemia
     (ii) Leptospirosis icterohaemorrhagiae (Weil's)
    (iii) Yellow fever
2. Drugs and toxins
      (i) Direct toxicity e.g. carbon tetrachloride
     (ii) Hypersensitivity e.g. penicillin
3. Hepatorenal syndrome
      Oliguria secondary to hepatic failure, usually following
      biliary tract surgery or cirrhosis
4. Haemolytic-uraemic syndrome
5. Incompatible blood transfusion
6. Toxaemia of pregnancy
7. Other causes of 'shock'

Further reading

Papper, S. & Vaamonde, C.A. (1971) *Diseases of the Kidney* 2nd edn., ed. Strauss, M.B. & Welt L.G. p. 1139 Boston: Little Brown.
Wilkinson, S.P. (1975) *Medicine,* 2nd series, **29,** 1647.

CAUSES OF POLYDIPSIA AND POLYURIA

1. *Decreased vasopressin production*
   (i) Cranial diabetes insipidus
       Congenital
       Head injury or neurosurgery
       Tumours e.g. craniopharyngioma
       Sarcoid, histiocytosis X, TB, etc.
   (ii) Psychogenic polydipsia
2. *Decreased renal tubular response to vasopressin*
   (i) Congenital nephrogenic DI
   (ii) Hypercalcaemia or hypokalaemia
   (iii) Chronic renal failure
   (iv) Obstructive uropathy
   (v) Lithium therapy
   (vi) Psychogenic polydipsia
3. *Osmotic diuresis*
   (i) Heavy glycosuria
   (ii) Mannitol therapy
4. *Dry mouth*
   Sjögren's syndrome

Further reading

Edwards, C.P.W. (1975) *Advanced Medicine, Symposium 11,* ed. Lant, A.F. p. 276. London: Pitman.

ARGININE VASOPRESSIN (Antidiuretic hormone)

Causes of inappropriate ADH secretion

1. *Neoplasm*
   Ectopic synthesis, especially bronchial oat-cell Ca.
2. *Neuro-hypophyseal disease*
   Intra-cranial inflammation, bleeding, tumour, trauma, etc.
3. *Non-neoplastic thoracic disease*
   TB, pneumonia, cardiac surgery
4. *Endocrine*
   Hypoadrenalism, hypothyroidism, hypopituitarism
5. *Drugs*
   Chlorpropamide
   Carbamazepine
   Cyclophosphamide
   Clofibrate
   Thiazides
6. *Miscellaneous*
   Pain, trauma, hypotension, leukaemia, lymphoma

Further reading

Bisset, G.W. & Jones, N.F. (1975) *Recent Advances in Renal Disease* ed. Jones, N.F., **1,** 396. Edinburgh: Churchill Livingstone.

Rheumatology

RAYNAUD'S PHENOMENON
Paroxysmal digital ischaemia, usually accompanied by pallor and cyanosis and followed by erythema

Causes
 1. *Reflex vasoconstriction*
    (i) Raynaud's disease
    (ii) Cervical spondylosis
    (iii) Shoulder-hand syndrome
    (iv) Vibrating machinery
 2. *Arterial occlusion*
    (i) Thoracic outlet syndromes (p. 161)
    (ii) Embolus, thrombosis or stenosis
    (iii) Arteriosclerosis
    (iv) Buerger's disease
    (v) Injury (Volkmann's ischaemia)
 3. *'Collagen vascular' disease*
    (i) Systemic sclerosis
    (ii) Polyarteritis
    (iii) SLE
    (iv) Rh. arthritis, Sjøgren's
 4. *Increased blood agglutination*
    (i) Cold agglutinins
    (ii) Dysproteinaemias
    (iii) Polycythaemia, leukaemia, Moschcowitz's, etc.
 5. *Neurological:* paralysis or disuse of a limb
 6. *Cold injury:* frost bite
 7. *Toxins*
    (i) Vinyl chloride
    (ii) Ergot
    (iii) Heavy metals
    (iv) Tobacco
 8. *Drugs:ß*-blockers
 9. *Malnutrition and cachexia*
10. *Miscellaneous rare causes*
    Typhoid fever, amyloidosis, myxoedema etc.

Further reading
Leading article (1972) *British Medical Journal,* **3,** 782.

Causes of cryoglobulinaemia
1. Idiopathic
2. Collagen-vascular disease
3. Infections
     Bacterial endocarditis
     Syphilis
     Infectious mononucleosis
     Cytomegalic virus infection
     Leprosy
     Kala-azar
     Toxoplasmosis
4. Multiple myeloma and Waldenstrøm's macroglobulinaemia
5. Myeloproliferative disease
6. Miscellaneous
     Sickle-cell disease
     Glomerulonephritis
     Myocardial infarction
     Ulcerative colitis
     Chronic liver disease, etc.

RHEUMATOID DISEASE
ARA criteria for diagnosis of rheumatoid arthritis
1. Morning stiffness
2. Pain and tenderness in at least one joint
3. Swelling of one joint for six weeks or more
4. Swelling in another joint
5. Symmetrical joint swelling
6. Subcutaneous nodules
7. Periarticular osteoporosis, bony erosions
8. Positive test for rheumatoid factor
9. Poor mucin precipitate of synovial fluid
10. Typical synovial histology
11. Typical nodule histology

Classical rheumatoid = 7 of above
Definite rheumatoid = 5 of above
Probable rheumatoid = 3 of above

Further reading

Bluestone, R. & Bacon, P.A. (1977) *Clinics in Rheumatic Diseases,* **3**, No. 3, Philadelphia: Saunders.
Katz, W.A. (1977) Rheumatic Diseases, Diagnosis & Management, p. 421, Philadelphia, Lippincott.

Complications of rheumatoid disease
1. *Poor general health*
    (i) Weight loss
    (ii) Anaemia
    (iii) Depression and social problems
2. *Joint complications*
    (i) Deformity, subluxation, etc.
    (ii) Pyoarthrosis
    (iii) Tendon rupture, due to attrition or nodules
    (iv) Nerve compression due to tenosynovial swelling
    (v) Cord or root compression, due to cervical subluxation
    (vi) Baker's synovial cyst
    (vii) Acute rupture of synovial sac, especially in knee
    (viii) Hoarseness, due to crico-arytenoid arthritis
    (ix) Deafness, due to arthritis of auditory ossicles
3. *Pressure sores and infected ulcers*
4. *Osteoporosis and muscle atrophy*
5. *Pulmonary*
    (i) Pleuritis, effusion
    (ii) Nodule in lung or pleura
    (iii) Fibrosing alveolitis
    (iv) Caplan's syndrome in pneumoconiosis
6. *Cardiac*
    (i) Pericarditis
    (ii) Rheumatoid granuloma of heart
7. *Ocular*
    (i) Scleritis
    (ii) Scleromalacia perforans
    (iii) Uveitis
    (iv) Sjøgren's syndrome
8. *Arteritis*
    (i) Digital ischaemia (may be Raynaud's)
    (ii) Leg ulcers
    (iii) Mesenteric ischaemia
    (iv) Arteritis of lungs, kidneys, liver, etc.
9. *Peripheral and autonomic neuropathy*
10. *Lymphadenopathy*
    Usually in region of an inflamed joint
11. *Amyloidosis*
    May develop renal vein thrombosis
12. *Felty's syndrome* (Splenomegaly, RA and leucopenia)
13. *Complications of therapy*
14. *Associated auto-immune disease*
    (i) Pernicious anaemia
    (ii) Thyroiditis
    (iii) Haemolytic anaemia, etc.
15. *Subfertility* (Prior to development of arthritis)

Further reading
Sheldon, P. (1975) *Medicine,* 2nd series, **15,** 693.

Factors in the anaemia of RA
1. Fe deficiency
    (i) GI blood loss due to drugs (aspirin, indomethacin, butazolidine, glucocorticoids)
    (ii) Defective Fe utilization ('anaemia of chronic disorders')
2. Folic acid deficiency
3. Marrow hypoplasia
4. Haemodilution
5. Haemolysis, especially in Felty's syndrome
6. Increased incidence of pernicious anaemia

Conditions in which rheumatoid factor may be present
1. Collagen vascular disease, especially Sjøgren's syndrome and rheumatoid disease
2. Infection
    (i) Syphilis
    (ii) Kala-azar
    (iii) Leprosy
    (iv) Infective endocarditis
    (v) Tuberculosis
    (vi) Rubella
    (vii) Infectious mononucleosis
3. Sarcoidosis
4. Asbestosis
5. Chronic liver disease
6. Post-blood transfusion
7. Malignancy
8. Waldenstrøm's macroglobulinaemia
9. Renal transplantation
10. Glomerulonephritis
11. Relatives of RA patients
12. Normal old age

Conditions associated with Sjøgren's syndrome
1. Collagen-vascular disease
2. Hashimoto's thyroiditis
3. Peripheral neuropathy
4. Renal tubular acidosis
5. Primary biliary cirrhosis
6. Diffuse interstitial pulmonary fibrosis
7. Cryoglobulinaemia
8. Hyperglobulinaemic purpura (Waldenstrøm)
9. Lymphoma
10. Pancreatitis

LUPUS ERYTHEMATOSUS
ARA Criteria for diagnosis of SLE
 1. Facial erythema
 2. Discoid lupus
 3. Raynaud's phenomenon
 4. Alopecia
 5. Photosensitivity
 6. Oral or nasopharyngeal ulceration
 7. Arthritis without deformity
 8. LE cells
 9. Chronic false positive WR
10. Profuse proteinuria
11. Cellular casts
12. Pleurisy or pericarditis
13. Haemolytic anaemia, leukopenia or thrombocytopenia
14. Psychosis or convulsions

The presence of four or more features strongly suggests SLE

Further reading

Cohen, A.S. et al (1971) *Bulletin of Rheumatic Diseases,* **21,** 643.

Conditions in which antinuclear antibodies may be present
 1. Collagen vascular disease, esp. SLE
 2. Chronic liver disease
 3. Hashimoto's thyroiditis, thymoma, myasthenia gravis
 4. Pernicious anaemia
 5. Tuberculosis
 6. Leprosy
 7. Diffuse pulmonary fibrosis
 8. Lymphoma or other malignancy
 9. Ulcerative colitis
10. Normal old people

Further reading

Holborow, E.J. (1978) *British Journal of Hospital Medicine,* **19,** 250.

Patterns of nuclear fluorescence

Pattern	Antigen	Found in:
Diffuse	DNA	SLE, rheumatoid and other collagen-vascular disease
Peripheral ('shaggy')	DNA	Active SLE with nephritis or vasculitis
Nucleolar	RNA	Mainly systemic sclerosis
Speckled	(i) SM RNA-ase resistant	Mainly SLE
	(ii) Extractable nuclear antigen RNA-ase sensitive	Mixed connective tissue disease

Further reading

Biundo, J.J. & Cummings, N.A. (1977) *Rheumatic Diseases, Diagnosis and Management,* ed. Katz, W.A. p. 269. Philadelphia: Lippincott.

Holborow, E.J. (1978) *British Journal of Hospital Medicine,* **19,** 250.

VASCULITIS

No satisfactory classification of vasculitis exists, since the clinical syndromes in many cases overlap and their pathogenesis is imperfectly understood.

Causes

1. *Polyarteritis nodosa and related disorders*
    (i) Polyarteritis nodosa
    (ii) Cranial arteritis
    (iii) Aortic arch syndrome (incl. Takayashu's)
    (iv) Polymyalgia rheumatica
    (v) Wegener's granuloma and lethal midline granuloma
    (vi) Allergic granulomatosis (Churg)
    (vii) Hypersensitivity (leukocytoclastic) angiitis (Zeek)
    (viii) Henoch-Schönlein purpura
2. *Rheumatic and collagen diseases*
    (i) Rheumatoid arthritis
    (ii) Sjøgren's
    (iii) Rheumatic fever
    (iv) SLE
    (v) Dermatomyositis
    (vi) Systemic sclerosis
3. *Endarteritis obliterans*
    (i) Any chronic ulcer, e.g. peptic ulcer, ulcerative colitis
    (ii) Syphilis
    (iii) TB
    (iv) Buerger's
4. *Infective*
    (i) Extension of perivascular inflammation: cellulitis, abscess, meningitis, etc.
    (ii) Septicaemia, septic emboli
    (iii) Cutaneous arteritis during rash of meningococcaemia, scarlatina, typhus fever, etc.
5. *Cutaneous vasculitis not included above:*
    (i) Some drug rashes
    (ii) Erythema multiforme
    (iii) Erythema nodosum
    (iv) Nodular vasculitis
    (v) Erythema induratum (Bazin)
    (vi) Erythema elevatum diutinum, etc.

Further reading

Ryan, T.J. (1973) *Advanced Medicine 9th Symposium,* ed. Walker, G., p. 319. London: Pitman.

Causes of hypermobile joints
1. Marfan's
2. Ehlers-Danlos
3. Osteogenesis imperfecta
4. Inflammatory polyarthritis, e.g. RA
5. Charcot's arthropathy
6. Homocystinuria
7. Hyperlysinaemia
8. Idiopathic

Causes of generalised stiffness
1. *Unaccustomed exercise*
2. *Systemic infection,* e.g. influenza
3. *Arthritis,* especially
     (i) Rheumatoid
    (ii) Polymyalgia rheumatica
   (iii) Generalised osteoarthrosis
    (iv) Ochronosis
     (v) Haemochromatosis
    (vi) Serum sickness
4. *Neuromuscular disease*
     (i) 'Stiff man syndrome' (tonic muscle rigidity)
    (ii) Cervical spondylosis with myelopathy
   (iii) Extrapyramidal disease
          Torsion dystonia
          Hepato-lenticular degeneration (Wilson's)
          Parkinsonism
    (iv) Tetanus
     (v) McArdle's myopathy
    (vi) Myotonia
   (vii) Dermatomyositis
5. *Scleroderma* (p. 168)
6. *Generalised oedema*
     (i) Anascara
    (ii) Scleroedema
   (iii) Erythroderma
7. *Hypothyroidism,* especially in cold weather
8. *Mucopolysaccharidoses* (p. 165)

The 'shoulder-hand syndrome' (Sudek's atrophy)

Associated conditions:
1. Myocardial infarction
2. Trauma
3. Cervical spinal lesion
4. Hemiplegia
5. Brain tumour
6. Epilepsy (? phenobarbitone)
7. Electro-convulsive therapy
8. Pulmonary lesions
9. Herpes zoster
10. Panniculitis
11. Vasculitis

Causes of carpal tunnel syndrome
1. Idiopathic
2. Pregnancy, 'Pill', pre-menstrual
3. Myxoedema
4. Acromegaly
5. Rheumatoid arthritis (may be presenting symptom)
6. Previous scaphoid fracture
7. Intermittent trauma
8. Mucopolysaccharidosis V (Scheie's syndrome)

Thoracic outlet syndromes
1. Scalenus anticus
2. Cervical rib
3. Hyperabduction
4. Costoclavicular
5. Clavipectoral
6. Postural and sleep syndromes

Radiological features of some arthropathies

Osteo-arthrosis
1. New bone formation
     Osteophytes
     Peri-articular ossicles
     Loose bodies
2. Cartilage loss, often confined to weight-bearing surface
3. Sclerosis and subchondral cavitation
4. Subluxation of hip, shoulder, terminal IP joints
5. **No** ankylosis

Gout
1. Punched-out erosions of joint margins
2. Erosions occur beyond joint capsule
3. Spotted appearance of carpals
4. Cartilage loss
5. **No** osteoporosis or new bone formation

Ankylosing spondylitis
1. Bilateral erosive SI disease, with later sclerosis
2. Erosion in intervertebral facets and costo-vertebral joints
3. Calcified spinal ligaments
4. Erosion in limb joints, especially hips
5. Irregularity of weight-bearing surfaces
6. Calcification of the entheses

Rheumatoid arthritis
1. Juxta-articular osteoporosis
2. Cartilage loss
3. Marginal and surface erosions
4. Subluxations, dislocations and carpal ankylosis
5. **No** sclerosis or new bone formation

Chondrocalcinosis
Calcium deposits (punctate-linear opacities) are seen esp. in AP view of knees, and in symphysis pubis and wrists.

Causes of a periosteal reaction
1. Osteomyelitis
2. Healing fracture
3. Rheumatoid arthritis (especially juvenile)
4. Hypertrophic pulmonary osteoarthropathy
5. Psoriatic arthritis
6. Reiter's syndrome
7. Cellulitis
8. Bone tumours, e.g. osteo-sarcoma
9. Subperiosteal haemorrhage e.g. scurvy
10. Polyarteritis nodosa

Conditions associated with ankylosing spondylitis
1. Aortic insufficiency
2. Uveitis
3. Pulmonary fibrosis
4. Amyloidosis
5. Enteropathy—Ulcerative colitis
                Crohn's disease
                Whipple's disease
6. Psoriasis
7. Reiter's disease

CAUSES OF HYPERURICAEMIA
1. **Increased purine synthesis**
    (i) Primary gout (in 25 per cent of cases)
    (ii) Lesch-Nyhan syndrome (Congenital mental deficiency, choreo-athetosis and lip chewing)
2. **Increased turnover of preformed purines**
    (i) Myeloproliferative disease and lymphoma
    (ii) Chronic haemolysis
    (iii) Psoriasis
    (iv) Fructose ingestion
    (v) High purine diet
3. **Decreased renal excretion**
    (i) Primary gout (in 75 per cent of cases)
    (ii) Chronic renal failure
    (iii) Hyperparathyroidism
    (iv) Lead nephropathy
    (v) Down's syndrome
    (vi) Increased organic acid production:
                Exercise
                Starvation, vomiting
                Diabetic keto-acidosis
                Alcohol   ·
                Toxaemia of pregnancy
                Glycogen storage disease (G6P deficiency)
                Hyperlipidaemia
    (vii) Drugs:
                Salicylates (in low dosage)
                Uricosurics (in low dosage)
                Diuretics
                Pyrazinamide
                Ethambutol

Se uric acid also tends to be high in patients with hypertension, obesity and high IQ

Further reading

Nuki, G. (1975) *Advanced Medicine, Symposium 11,* ed. Lant, A.F. p. 334. London: Pitman.

CALCIUM PYROPHOSPHATE ARTHROPATHY

Pseudogout (chondrocalcinosis) may mimic gout, rheumatoid arthritis, osteoarthrosis or neuropathic arthropathy
Numerous intraleucocytic crystals (CPPD) in synovial fluid are diagnostic

ASSOCIATED CONDITIONS

1. Metabolic
  Hyperuricaemia (with or without gout)
  Hyperparathyroidism
  Paget's disease of bone
  Hepato-lenticular degeneration (Wilson's)
  Haemochromatosis
  Acromegaly
  Ochronosis
  Hypophosphatasia
  Diabetes mellitus

2. Hypertension or atheroma

3. Renal failure or calculi

4. Secondary to other arthropathies
  Osteoarthrosis
  Neuropathic arthropathy
  Rheumatoid arthritis

5. Idiopathic

Further reading

Yu, T. & Katz, W.A. (1977) *Rheumatic Diseases, Diagnosis and Management,* ed. Katz, W.A. p. 724, Philadelphia: Lippincott.
McCarty, D.J. et al. (1976) *Arthritis and Rheumatism,* **19,** 275 to 500.

INHERITED DISORDERS OF CONNECTIVE TISSUE
A. Defect in fibrous elements
1. *Primary disorder of biosynthesis of CT*
    (i) Ehlers-Danlos syndromes (at least 7 types)
    (ii) Osteogenesis imperfecta (deficiency of Type I collagen)
    (iii) Marfan syndrome (at least 4 types)
2. *Secondary damage to CT*
    (i) Alkaptonuria (defective homogentisic acid degradation)
    (ii) Homocystinuria (resembles the Marfan syndrome, but with thromboses and osteoporosis; due to a specific enzyme defect)
    (iii) Menkes' 'kinky hair' syndrome (defective copper transport)
    (iv) Pseudo-xanthoma elasticum (degeneration of elastic fibres)

B. Mucopolysaccharidoses
Lysosomal storage diseases with disordered glycosaminoglycan degradation due to specific enzyme deficiencies

Type	Clinical features
I *Hurler*	Gargoylism, dwarfing, hepatosplenomegaly, mental deficiency, corneal opacity, deafness. Death in childhood.
II *Hunter*	A milder form, limited to males
III *Sanfilippo**	Severe CNS changes, minor somatic changes.
IV *Morquio*	Characteristic skeletal changes (dwarfing, knock-knee, barrel chest, etc), normal I.Q.
V *Scheie**	Stiff joints, coarse facies, corneal opacity.
VI *Maroteaux**	Similar to Hurler's but normal I.Q.
VII *Dygvve**	Similar to Morquio's but mentally retarded

Very rare

Further reading
McKusick, V.A. (1976) *Advanced Medicine* ed. Peters, D.K. Symposium. 12, p. 170. London: Pitman.

Causes of a positive WR
1. Infections
    (i) Syphilis or yaws
    (ii) Occasionally after vaccinia, infective hepatitis, infectious mononucleosis, mycoplasma, malaria, leprosy, trypanosomiasis, etc.
2. Collagen-vascular disease, esp. SLE and Sjøgren's disease
3. Auto-immune thyroiditis (Hashimoto's)
4. Auto-immune haemolytic anaemia
5. Dysproteinaemia
6. Narcotic addiction
7. Normal old age

The administration of penicillin to patients with a chronic biological false positive reaction (BFP) may be dangerous because of their increased risk of hypersensitivity.

Further reading

Catterall, R.D. (1973) *Advanced Medicine, 9th. Symposium,* ed. Walker, G., p. 97. London: Pitman.

Dermatology

SKIN CHANGES ASSOCIATED WITH SYSTEMIC MALIGNANCY

A. **Genetic syndromes predisposing to neoplasm**
 1. Phakomatoses (Disseminated hamartomata of eye, skin and brain)
    - (i) Neurofibromatosis (von Recklinghausen's)
    - (ii) Epiloia (Bourneville's, tuberose sclerosis)
    - (iii) Basal cell naevoid syndrome (Gorlin's)
    - (iv) Cerebellar haemangioblastoma (von Hippel-Lindau)
    - (v) Encephalotrigeminal angiomatosis (Sturge-Weber's)
 2. Familial tylosis (keratoderma) and Ca oesophagus
 3. Familial polyposis coli (Gardner's) with sebaceous cysts
 4. Defective immunosurveillance
    - (i) Wiskott-Aldrich
    - (ii) Ataxia telangiectasia
    - (iii) Chediak-Higashi
 5. Small intestinal polyposis with perioral lentigines (Peutz-Jegher's syndrome). Rarely associated with carcinoma
 6. Multiple endocrine adenomatosis (Type 2) with pigmentation, mucosal neuromas and medullary Ca thyroid (p. 137)
 7. Werner's premature ageing syndrome
 8. Cowden's disease. Warty papules on face, oral mucosa and hands antedating Ca of breast, thyroid or female reproductive tract

B. **Signs of exposure to a carcinogen**
 1. Nicotine staining of fingers
 2. Signs of arsenic ingestion
    - (i) Keratoses
    - (ii) Diffuse pigmentation with 'rain-drops' of paler normal skin
 3. Bowen's disease of covered skin
 4. X-ray dermatitis or multiple basal cell ca. over spine may indicate increased risk of leukaemia

C. **Direct involvement of skin by malignancy**
 1. Direct spread, e.g. carcinoma erysipeloides or carcinoma telangiectoides
 2. Metastases
 3. Paget's disease of skin (nipple or perineum)
 4. Leukaemic infiltrate
 5. Skin changes of lymphoma
    - (i) Prelymphomatous poikiloderma
    - (ii) Cutaneous spread of a systemic lymphoma
    - (iii) Mycosis fungoides and Sezary's syndrome

(contd.)

D. Other associations
  1. Pigmentation
  2. Pallor
  3. Pruritis (esp. lymphoma)
  4. Acanthosis nigricans and papillomatosis (esp. GI malignancy)
  5. Dermatomyositis
  6. Hypertrophic pulmonary osteo-arthropathy (p. 34)
  7. Herpes zoster (esp. lymphoma)
  8. Acquired ichthyosis (esp. lymphoma)
  9. Figurate erythema, e.g. Erythema gyratum repens
 10. Rapid onset of multiple basal-cell papillomata (Leser-Trelat)
 11. Hypertrichosis lanuginosa (acquired)
 12. Widespread viral infection (eczema herpeticum, etc.) due to immune paresis of malignancy
 13. Lymphoedema due to lymphatic obstruction by malignancy
 14. Generalised hyperhidrosis
 15. Necrolytic migratory erythema of glucagonoma
 16. Nodular panniculitis (esp. Ca pancreas)
 17. Superficial migratory thrombophebitis (esp. Ca pancreas)
 18. Flush and telangiectasia of malignant carcinoid
 19. Bullous pyoderma of leukaemia
 20. Bullous eruptions e.g. pemphigoid (controversial)

Further reading
Sneddon, I.B.(1963) *British Medical Journal,* **2,** 405.

SCLERODERMA
Scleroderma refers to sclerosis (induration) of the skin and subcutaneous tissue, but some authorities restrict the term to morphoea and systemic sclerosis, and use the term pseudoscleroderma for sclerosis due to other causes

Causes of scleroderma
  1. Systemic sclerosis or morphoea
  2. Dermatomyositis, LE or rheumatoid disease
  3. Cutaneous porphyria
  4. Vinyl chloride exposure
  5. Chronic gravitational oedema
  6. Chronic scurvy (esp. legs)
  7. Carcinoid syndrome
  8. Mucinous infiltration
       (i) diffuse myxoedema
      (ii) lichen myxoedematosus
     (iii) scleroedema of Buschke
  9. Werner's progeria
 10. Graft-versus-host reaction
 11. Eosinophilic fasciitis

PORPHYRIA

Simplified synthetic pathway of haem

Key: ALA = amino-laevulinic acid
PBG = porphobilinogen
UP = uroporphyrin
CP = corproporphyrin
PP = protoporphyrin

HEPATIC PORPHYRIAS

A. Genetic autosomal dominant

1. *Acute intermittent porphyria (AIP)*
Classical triad of dark urine, abdominal pain and neuropsychiatric symptoms. May be nausea, constipation, tachycardia, electrolyte disturbances and pigmentation but *no* frank photosensitivity
Acute attacks precipitated by drugs (barbiturates, sulphonamides, choloroquine, oestrogen and griseofulvin)

Lab.
  (i) Urine darkens on standing and may fluoresce pink under UV radiation
  (ii) Watson-Schwartz Test +ve
    2 ml. urine + 2ml. Ehrlich's aldehyde reagent + 4 ml saturated sodium acetate soln. A purple colour is due to *porphobilinogen* or urobilinogen, but urobilinogen is soluble in chloroform
  (iii) Urinary ALA and PBG are markedly increased, but porphyrins are normal or only slightly increased

2. *Porphyria variegata*
Clinical features of both AIP and PCT

3. *Hereditary coproporphyria*
Rare, resembles AIP

(contd.)

B. Porphyria cutanea tarda
(PCT, 'symptomatic' porphyria)
Photosensitivity, skin fragility, pigmentation and hirsutism

Causes
1. Idiosyncratic response to liver damage, esp. alcohol-induced
2. Dose-related response to toxins, e.g. hexachlorobenzene (a wheat fungicide)
3. Porphyrin-producing hepatic neoplasm

Lab.
  (i) Urine fluoresces pink, due to increased UP III and CP III
  (ii) Faecal CP III increased
  (iii) Raised Se iron

ERYTHROPOIETIC PORPHYRIAS
1. Congenital erythropoietic porphyria (Gunther's disease)
Very rare defect in haem synthesis characterised by pink teeth, hypertrichosis and severe photosensitivity leading to multilating ulceration. May be haemolytic anaemia and splenomegaly

2. Erythrohepatic proto-porphyria
(Formerly called erythropoietic proto-porphyria)
A familial syndrome with a variety of photosensitivity changes, and burning pain characteristically relieved by cold running water. Also superficial linear scars (pseudorhagades)

Lab.
  (i) Erythrocyte PP is invariably increased
  (ii) Urinary porphyrins normal

Diagnosis of the porphyrias
Remember that:
1. In an acute porphyric attack, the fresh urine may be normal colour and non-fluorescent
2. Urine tests are unreliable for the detection of cutaneous porphyrias, and examination of blood and faeces is necessary

Causes of coproporphyrinuria other than porphyria
1. Alcohol abuse
2. Lead poisoning
3. Liver disease or biliary obstruction
4. Lymphoma, pernicious anaemia, infectious mononucleosis

Further reading
Brodie, M.J. *et al* (1977), *Lancet,* **2,** 699.
Pimstone, N.R. (1975) *Modern Trends in Gastroenterology,* ed. Read, A.E. Vol. 5, p. 373. London: Butterworth.

LIPOPROTEINS
Electrophoretic strip:

chylomicrons—cleared from plasma by
lipoprotein lipase

ß-lipoproteins (low density lipoprotein—LDL)
carry cholesterol

pre-ß-lipoproteins (very low density
lipoprotein—VLDL) carry endogenously
synthesised glycerides

α-lipoproteins (high density lipoprotein—HDL)
take up cholesterol for excretion via liver

Hyperlipoproteinaemia (Fredrickson's classification)
Type 1. Familial hyperchylomicronaemia
Presents in childhood as severe hyperlipaemia. Very rare

Type 2. Hyperbeta-lipoproteinaemia of normal density
May be primary (familial hypercholesterolaemia) or secondary to
myxoedema, cholestasis or nephrotic syndrome

Type 3. Hyperbeta-lipoproteinaemia of low density
Usually genetic

Type 4. Hyperprebeta-lipoproteinaemia
A common abnormality secondary to metabolic disease such as
diabetes mellitus, obesity, alcoholism, pancreatitis and nephrotic
syndrome

Type 5. 'Mixed'
Increased chylomicrons and pre-ß-lipoproteins

Clinical presentation of hyperlipidaemia
1. Ischaemic heart disease
2. Peripheral atheroma
3. Xanthoma
4. Gout
5. Tendinitis
6. Aortic stenosis

Clinical types of xanthomas

1. Plane   — in palm creases and eyelids (xanthelasma)
2. Tendon   — nodules attached to tendons or ligaments
3. Tuberous — larger lesions which may be tender
4. Eruptive — multiple small lesions occurring in 'showers',
                 often with a red halo

(contd.)

Palmar crease xanthoma suggests either cholestasis or Type 3
Xanthelasma suggests Type 2, but can occur in normal people

Tangier disease
HDL is defective and cholesterol accumulates in reticuloendothelial
tissues.

Further reading

Lewis, B. (1976) *The Hyperlipidaemias* Oxford: Blackwell
Lewis, B. (1975) *Medicine,* 2nd series, **14,** 668.

CAUSES OF PHOTOSENSITIVITY
1. *Circulating photosensitisers*
   - (i) Porphyria (p. 170)
   - (ii) Drugs
     - Phenothiazines
     - Diuretics
     - Oral antidiabetics
     - Tetracyclines (esp. demethylchlortetracycline)
     - Nalidixic acid
     - Sulphonamides
2. *Contact photosensitisers*
   - (i) Tar products
   - (ii) Furocoumarins (perfumes and plants)
   - (iii) Chemicals in soaps and bleaches
3. *Idiopathic dermatoses*
   - (i) Photosensitive eczema and actinic reticuloid
   - (ii) Polymorphic light eruption
   - (iii) Hydroa vacciniforme
   - (iv) Solar urticaria
4. *Lack of protection from UVR* (decreased melanin in skin)
   - (i) Albinism and vitiligo
   - (ii) Phenylketonuria
   - (iii) Hypopituitarism
5. *Metabolic defect*
   - (i) Pellagra
   - (ii) Hartnup disease
6. *Rare congenital diseases*
e.g. Xeroderma pigmentosum, poikiloderma congenitale, etc.

UVR may also precipitate or exacerbate other dermatoses such as
LE, herpes simplex and rosacea

PIGMENTATION

CAUSES OF DIFFUSE HYPERPIGMENTATION
1. **Congenital**
   (i) Racial or genetic
   (ii) Fanconi's syndrome (pancytopenia with multiple congenital defects)
2. **Physical agents**
   (i) Radiation e.g. UVR
   (ii) Chronic rubbing e.g. 'vagabond's itch'
3. **Post-inflammatory** e.g. erythroderma
4. **Endocrine**
   (i) Pregnancy, oral contraceptives
   (ii) Hypoadrenalism
   (iii) Acromegaly
   (iv) Hyperthyroidism
   (v) Phaeochromocytoma
   (vi) ACTH therapy or ectopic ACTH from carcinoma
5. **Cachexia of any cause** (esp. malignancy)
6. **Chronic infection**
   Especially malaria, kala-azar, TB, bacterial endocarditis
7. **Nutritional deficiency**
   (i) Malabsorption (esp. sprue)
   (ii) Isolated A, C, B_{12} or folate deficiency
   (iii) Pellagra
8. **Hepatic disease** (esp. biliary cirrhosis, haemochromatosis and hepatolenticular degeneration)
9. **Chronic renal failure**
10. **Collagen-vascular disease**
    (i) Systemic sclerosis
    (ii) Juvenile RA (Still's)
    (iii) Dermatomyositis
    (iv) SLE
11. **Cutaneous porphyria**
12. **Drugs and chemicals**
    (i) Arsenicals
    (ii) Busulphan
    (iii) ACTH
    (iv) Oestrogens
    (v) Chlorpromazine
    (vi) Chloroquine
    (vii) Photodynamic agents e.g. psoralens
13. **Pigmentation not due to melanin**
    (i) Jaundice—yellow
    (ii) Carotenaemia—yellow
    (iii) Mepacrine—yellow
    (iv) Ochronosis (alkaptanuria)—blue-black
    (v) Argyria (due to silver)—slate-grey
    (vi) Chrysiasis (due to gold)—blue-grey
    (vii) Haemosiderosis (due to iron)—red-brown

CAUSES OF HYPOMELANOSIS (MELANIN DEFICIENCY)

A. Circumscribed depigmented patches

Congenital
1. Piebaldism (partial albinism)
2. Waardenburg's syndrome (characteristic facies, with deafness and a white forelock)
3. Tuberose sclerosis (epiloia)
4. Naevus depigmentosus

Acquired
1. Post-inflammatory
     (i) Pityriasis alba
     (ii) Eczema, esp. in Negro
     (iii) Scarring, e.g. burns, varicella
2. Infection
     (i) Pityriasis versicolor
     (ii) Pinta
     (iii) Leprosy
3. Immunological
     (i) Vitiligo
     (ii) Halo naevus (with circulating anti-melanoma antibody)
     (iii) Malignant melanoma
4. Toxins
     (i) Hydroquinones
     (ii) Phenolic germicides

B. Generalized diffuse hypomelanosis

Congenital
1. Albinism
2. Phenylketonuria
3. Chediak-Higashi syndrome

Acquired
Hypopituitarism

Further reading

Bleehan, S.S. (1974) *Advanced Medicine, Symposium 10,* ed. Ledingham, J.G.G. p. 317, London: Pitman.

Conditions associated with vitiligo
1. Organ-specific auto-immune disease
     (i) Thyroiditis
     (ii) Adrenalitis
     (iii) Pernicious anaemia
     (iv) Juvenile-onset diabetes mellitus
2. Alopecia areata
3. Morphoea
4. Halo naevus (Sutton's naevus)
5. Malignant melanoma
6. Sunburn and skin cancer

HIRSUTISM

Growth in the female of coarse terminal hair in the male adult
sexual pattern.

CAUSES

1. Idiopathic
A heterogenous group which includes racial and familial variation.
In some cases there is excessive androgen production, usually
ovarian, but sometimes adrenal.

2. Ovarian diseases
  (i) Polycystic ovaries
      The full Stein-Leventhal syndrome (obesity, amenorrhoea,
      sterility, polycystic ovaries but no virilization) is relatively
      rare, but partial forms are much commoner
  (ii) Postmenopausal ovarian stromal hyperplasia
  (iii) Ovarian hilus-cell hyperplasia
  (iv) Ovarian virilizing tumours (p. 127)
  (v) Gonadal dysgenesis
  (vi) Achard-Thiers syndrome
      Uniform obesity, hirsutism, hypertension and diabetes with
      normal adrenal function

3. Adrenal disease
  (i) ACTH-dependant cortical hyperplasia
      Cushing's
      Ectopic ACTH syndrome
  (ii) Adrenal tumours
  (iii) Late-onset congenital adrenal hyperplasia (C21 or 11β-
      hydroxylase defect)

4. Androgenic drugs
  Anabolic steroids
  Progestogens

Further reading
Givens, J.R. (1976) *Advances in Internal Medicine,* **21,** 221
London, D.R. (1974) *Advanced Medicine, Symposium 10,* ed.
Ledingham, J.G.G. p. 122. London: Pitman.

HYPERTRICHOSIS
Excessive hair growth in any site

Causes of generalised hypertrichosis
1. Cachexia, especially in children
2. Hereditary diseases
   e.g. erythrohepatic porphyria
   epidermolysis bullosa
   Cornelia de Lange syndrome
   trisomy E
   Hurler's syndrome
3. Head injury, especially in children
4. Dermatomyositis
5. Drugs
   (i) Phenytoin
   (ii) Glucocorticoids
   (iii) Diazoxide
6. Hypertrichosis lanuginosa
   This may be congenital or secondary to internal malignancy

Further reading

Rook, A. (1972) *Textbook of Dermatology,* 2nd edn. ed. Rook, A.
Wilkinson, D.S. & Ebling, F.J.G. p. 1575. Oxford: Blackwell

NAILS
Causes of white bands in the nails
1. Fungal infection
2. Chronic hypoalbuminaemia
3. Renal failure
4. Hodgkin's lymphoma
5. Sickle-cell disease
6. Malaria or leprosy
7. Toxins—cytotoxic drugs, arsenic
8. Darier's disease (longitudinal)
9. Congenital leukonychia

Causes of blue or black bands in the nails
1. Subungual haematoma
2. Melanoma
3. Infection by Candida or Pseudomonas
4. Drugs—Chloroquine, cytotoxics
5. Hepatolenticular degeneration (blue lunulae)

Further reading

Samman, P.D. (1972) *Textbook of Dermatology* end edn. ed. Rook,
A. Wilkinson, D.S., & Ebling, F.J.G.; p. 1642 Oxford: Blackwell.

CLINICAL PATTERNS OF DRUG ERUPTIONS

1. *Exanthemata* (scarlatiniform, morbilliform, papular, etc.)
   Barbiturates, antibiotics, chloral hydrate, etc.
2. *Urticaria*
   Penicillin, salicylates, etc.
3. *Exfoliative dermatitis* (erythroderma)
   Barbiturates, arsenicals, heavy metals, etc.
4. *Fixed eruptions*
   Barbiturates, sulphonamides, phenolphthalein
5. *Bullous eruptions*
   (i) Bromides, iodides, barbiturates, etc.
   (ii) Erythema multiforme (including Stevens-Johnson syndrome) and toxic epidermal necrolysis
   Sulphonamides, barbiturates, etc.
   (iii) Pemphigus, Penicillamine
6. *Purpura*
   (i) Drugs causing aplastic anaemia (p. 72)
   (ii) Selective thrombocytopenia: Sedormid, quinine
   (iii) Vascular: carbromal, glucocorticoids, penicillin, etc.
7. *Photo-sensitivity* (toxicity or allergy) (p. 173)
8. *Erythema nodosum*
   Sulphonamides
9. *Acneiform*
   Glucocorticoids, androgens, iodides, bromides, INAH, anticonvulsants, cyanocobalamin
10. *Lichenoid*
    Antimalarials, chlorothiazide, amiphenazole, gold
11. *Pigmentation* (p. 174)
12. *Hypertrichosis* (p. 177) *or hirsutism* (p. 176)
13. *Ichthyosis*
    Nicotinic acid, triparanol
14. *Eczema*
    Systemic administration of a drug after allergic contact dermatitis to the drug has developed
15. *Seborrhoeic dermatitis*
    Methyldopa
16. *SLE-like syndrome*
    Procainamide, hydrallazine, hydantoins, sulphonamides, etc.
17. *Psoriasiform*
    Practolol (also causes eye lesions, otitis media, sclerosing peritonitis, pleurisy and pericarditis)
18. Livedo reticularis. Amantadine
19. *Exacerbation of pre-existing skin disease*
    Porphyria—sulphonamides, barbiturates, chloroquine, oestrogens, griseofulvin
    Psoriasis—chloroquine, lithium

PRURITUS
Systemic causes of generalised pruritus
1. *Hepatic*
    Obstructive jaundice
    Recurrent pruritus of pregnancy
2. *Chronic renal failure* (may be due to secondary hyperparathyroidism)
3. *Blood*
    Malignant lymphoma
    Myeloproliferative disorders (p. 78)
    Fe-deficiency
    Mastocytosis
4. *Carcinoma,* especially lung, stomach, colon, breast
5. *Endocrine*
    Myxoedema or hyperthyroidism
    Carcinoid
6. *Drugs*
    Cocaine, morphine, stilbamidine
    Allergic drug reactions
7. *Parasites:* roundworm, trichiniasis, onchoceriasis, etc.
8. *Neurological*
    Tabes or GPI
    Multiple sclerosis
9. *Psychogenic*

Causes of severe pruritus due to skin disease
1. Mites (including scabies), insect bites, pediculosis
2. Eczema
3. Urticaria
4. Lichen planus
5. Dermatitis herpetiformis
6. Lichen simplex chronicus
7. Miliaria rubra (prickly heat)

Causes of palmar erythema
1. Dermatoses, e.g.
    eczema,
    tinea
    psoriasis
    pityriasis rubra pilaris

2. Increased oestrogens
    (i) Pregnancy
    (ii) Cirrhosis, especially alcoholic
3. Arthritis, especially rheumatoid
4. Shoulder-hand syndrome
5. Polycythaemia
6. Beri-beri
7. Mitral insufficiency
8. Diabetes mellitus

INDUSTRIAL SKIN DISEASES

1. **Contact dermatitis**
    (i) Due to irritants
        e.g. cutting oils
            caustics
            organic solvents
            detergents
            fibreglass
            physical factors, etc.
    (ii) Due to allergies
        e.g. chromate in cement, anti-rust paint, leather, etc.
            cobalt in cutting tools, polyester paints, etc.
            nickel in coins, jewellery, cleansing fluids, etc.
            epoxy resins in plastics, electrical components, etc.
            rubber chemicals (vulcanisers, accelerants and
            antioxidants) in tyres, hoses, couplings, etc.
2. **Leukoderma (depigmentation)**
    Due to hydroquinone derivatives e.g. in adhesives
3. **Industrial acne**
        (i)Folliculitis due to mineral oils
        (ii)Chloracne due to halogenated hydrocarbons
            e.g. dioxin
4. **Skin cancer**
    Due to chronic exposure to tar, mineral oils or chloroprene
5. **Scleroderma** (p. 168)
    Vinyl chloride disease (also causes Raynaud's, pulmonary
    fibrosis, acro-osteolysis and hepatic angio-sarcoma)
6. **Porphyria cutanea tarda**
    Due to dioxin
7. **Fluoride spots**
    Pigmented spots due to atmospheric fluoride from aluminium
    smelting
8. **Lichen planus**
    Due to colour film developers
9. **Chrome ulcers**

Further reading

Rycroft, R.J.G. & Calnan, C.D. (1976) *British Journal of Hospital Medicine*, **15**, 457.

PRESENTATION OF GONORRHOEA
1. **Primary genital infection**
    (i) Asymptomatic 'contact'
    (ii) Urethritis
    (iii) Vaginitis or cervicitis
2. **Extension of infection within genital tract**
    Female: endometritis, salpingitis, cystitis, etc.
    Male: prostatitis, cystitis, epididymitis, etc.
3. **Extra-genital dissemination**
    (i) Bacteraemia, may produce rigors or may be asymptomatic
    (ii) Arthritis-dermatitis syndrome:
        Papulo-pustular rash
        Tenosynovitis
        Arthralgia
        Myalgia
        Pyrexia
    (iii) Mono-articular septic joint
    (iv) Endocarditis, myocarditis or pericarditis
    (v) Hepatitis or peri-hepatitis
    (vi) Meningitis
    (vii) Pelvic peritonitis (in female)
4. **Primary extra-genital infection**
    (i) Conjunctivitis or ophthalmitis in neonates
    (ii) Skin infection, stomatitis, pharyngitis, proctitis, etc.
5. **Complications of the above**
    e.g. sterility after salpingitis
        stricture after urethritis

SECONDARY SYPHILIS
Clinical features
  1. Tiredness, fever, myalgia, sore throat and headache (often worst at night)
  2. Slight lymphadenopathy
  3. A polymorphous maculo-papular rash. Commonly involves palms and soles and is rarely irritable or vesicular.
  4. Condyloma lata of anus and genitalia
  5. Mucous patches of mouth, pharynx or larynx
  6. Patchy alopecia ('glades in the wood')
  7. Less commonly hepatitis, iritis, arthritis, periostitis or neuritis may occur

N.B. Must be considered in any atypical dermatosis

REITER'S SYNDROME
Clinical features
1. Non-specific urethritis, haematuria, sterile pyuria
2. Recurrent conjunctivitis or uveitis
3. Symmetrical subacute arthritis, tenosynovitis, periostitis
4. Circinate balanitis
5. Buccal ulcers
6. Keratoderma blenorrhagica, nail dystrophy
7. Plantar fasciitis

STEVENS-JOHNSON SYNDROME
Clinical features
1. Constitutional symptoms and high fever
2. Oral bullae and haemorrhagic crusting
3. Conjunctivitis, corneal ulcers, uveitis
4. Maculo-papular or bullous erythema multiforme
5. Urethritis, balanitis, vulvo-vaginitis
6. Bronchitis, pneumonitis
7. Renal lesions, diarrhoea, polyarthritis, otitis media, etc.

BEHCET'S SYNDROME
Clinical features
1. Buccal ulcers with a red areola
2. Conjunctivitis or uveitis
3. Cutaneous pustules, dermal nodules
4. Genital ulcers
5. CNS lesions: meningo-encephalitis, brain-stem syndromes, etc.
6. Thrombophlebitis
7. Rarely cardiac and pulmonary lesions

Immunology

Allergy means the specifically altered state of reactivity of a host following exposure to an allergen. The term applies to either hypersensitivity or immunity

Classification of harmful allergic reactions

Type I. Anaphylactic

▲ Antigen (Ag)
< Antibody (Ab)

Reaginic Ab (IgE) bound to tissue cells (e.g. mast cells) causes release of vasoactive substances on contact with Ag
Examples:
(i) Anaphylaxis
(ii) Hay-fever, urticaria, asthma

Type II. Cytotoxic

Ab (usually IgG or IgM) reacts with Ag bound to cell surface. This often involves complement fixation and cell damage
Examples:
  (i) Blood transfusion reactions
 (ii) Haemolytic disease of the newborn
(iii) Auto-allergic haemolytic anaemia
(iv) Post-streptococcal glomerulonephritis

Type III. Circulating immune complex (Arthus)

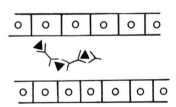

Free Ag and Ab combine and in certain conditions the complexes precipitate, with complement fixation and damage to small bloodvessels
Example: Serum sickness

Type IV: Cell-mediated (Delayed hypersensitivity)

Sensitised lymphocytes react with Ag deposited at a local site and release lymphokines such as mitogenic factor and macrophage migration inhibition factor. Probably involves cooperation between T and B lymphocytes and macrophages

Examples:
  (i) Skin reactions of the tuberculin type
  (ii) Homograft rejection
  (iii) Contact dermatitis
  (iv) Some auto-allergic diseases

T AND B LYMPHOCYTES
Distinctions between T and B lymphocytes

	T cells	B cells
Ig on cell surface	Absent or not easily demonstrated	Easily demonstrated
Fc receptors	Absent	Present
Complement receptors	Absent	Present
Sheep RBC binding to form rosettes	Yes	No
Response to mitogens—		
Phytohaemaglutinin	Yes	No
Conconavilin-A	Yes	No

Further reading
McConnell, I (1976) *Advanced Medicine Symposium 12,* ed. Peters, D.K. p. 1. London: Pitman.

B LYMPHOCYTE DEFICIENCIES

A. Primary

Hypogammaglobulinaemia
1. Congenital sex-linked (Bruton's)
2. Non-sex-linked agammaglobulinaemia
3. Hypogammaglobulinaemia of late onset
4. Combined immunodeficiency syndromes
    (i) Alymphocytic (Swiss-type)
    (ii) Thymic dysplasia
    (iii) Achondroplastic

Dysgammaglobulinaemia (normal γ-globulin on electrophoresis)
Types I to VII, e.g. selective deficit of IgA (Type IV) occurs in ataxia
telangiectasia, and selective deficit of IgM (Type V) in Wiskott-
Aldrich syndrome

B. Secondary

1. *Defective synthesis*
    (i) Prematurity or delayed maturity
    (ii) Lymphoma, myelomatosis or Waldenstrom's
        macroglobulinaemia
    (iii) Marrow disorders e.g. myelosclerosis, metastases,
        hypoplasia
    (iv) Irradiation and cytotoxic drugs
2. *Protein deficiency*
    (i) Nephrotic syndrome
    (ii) Protein-losing enteropathy
    (iii) Severe malnutrition or malabsorption
    (iv) Exfoliative dermatitis
    (v) Myotonic dystrophy

Causes of hypergammaglobulinaemia

1. *Diffuse 'broad band' type* (polyclonal gammopathy)
    (i) Chronic infection
    (ii) Hepatic disease
    (iii) 'Collagen vascular' disease, also ulcerative colitis, Crohn's,
        Hashimoto's thyroiditis, etc.
2. *Narrow 'M band' type* (monoclonal gammopathy)
    (i) Multiple myeloma
    (ii) Waldenstrom's macroglobulinaemia
    (iii) 'Benign' paraproteinaemia, especially in old people
    (iv) Heavy chain disease (Franklin's) (May be γ μ or α)
    (v) Bence-Jones proteinuria in absence of myelomatosis
    (vi) Leukaemia, lymphoma or carcinoma
    (vii) Primary cold agglutinins
    (viii) Amyloidosis
    (ix) Lichen myxoedematosus

T LYMPHOCYTE DEFICIENCIES
A. Primary
1. Thymic and parathyroid aplasia (Di George's)
2. Lymphopenia with normal immunoglobulins (Nezelof's)
3. Episodic lymphopenia with lymphocytotoxin
4. Qualitative lymphocyte defects (e.g. chronic mucocutaneous Candidiasis)

B. Secondary
1. Malignancy, esp. T cell lymphoma
2. Various (? immunological) diseases, e.g. eczema, multiple sclerosis
3. Kwashiorkor
4. Secondary to B cell deficiency

Further reading
Hobbs, J.R. (1974) *Blood and its Disorders*. ed. Hardisty, R. M. & Weatherall, D.J. p. 1319. Oxford: Blackwell
Hayward, A. (1975) *Immunology in Medical Practice* ed. Taylor, G. p. 33. London: Saunders.

CAUSES OF PHAGOCYTE DYSFUNCTION
1. Defective chemotaxis
    (i) Diabetes mellitus
    (ii) Steroid therapy
    (iii) Granulomata (Sarcoid, Crohn's)
    (iv) Some antibiotics, esp. tetracycline
    (v) Lazy leucocyte syndrome
2. Defective opsonisation
    (i) Complement deficiency e.g. C3 or C5
    (ii) IgM deficiency (e.g. in neonates)
    (iii) Sickle-cell anaemia
3. Defective intracellular bacterial killing
    (i) Chronic granulomatous disease of childhood
        Lymphadenopathy, hepatomegaly, pneumonia, dermatitis, abscesses, osteomyelitis. Due to defective hydrogen peroxide production
    (ii) Job's syndrome
        Recurrent cold staphylococcal abscesses
    (iii) Chediak-Higashi syndrome
        Partial oculo-cutaneous albinism. Giant lysosomes in granulocytes. Recurrent bacterial infections, sometimes with a lymphomatoid reaction
    (iv) Myeloperoxidase deficiency
    (v) Severe glucose-6-P dehydrogenase deficiency
    (vi) Drugs
        Glucocorticoids colchicine, etc.

Further reading
Baehner, R.L. (1972) *Paediatric Clinics of N. America,* **19**, 935.

COMPLEMENT
SOME INHERITED COMPLEMENT DEFECTS ASSOCIATED WITH
CLINICAL EFFECTS

Deficiency	Association
C1 inhibitor	Hereditary angio-oedema, due to unrestrained complement activation
C1r C1s	SLE-like syndrome
C2	'Immune-complex' disease Henoch-Schönlein purpura, glomerulonephritis, SLE, etc.
C3	Recurrent infections
Terminal components, C5–C9	Recurrent infections (esp. Neisseria)

Further reading
Lachmann, P.J. (1976) *Advanced Medicine,* ed. Peters, D.K. Vol. 12, p. 43. London: Pitman.

Skin testing for immunological reactions
Type I *(Prick test)* an urticarial wheal, developing within 20 minutes and resolving within 2 hours
Type III *(ID injection)* an ill-defined red swelling, sometimes purpuric, developing over several hours, maximal at 5–7 hours and resolving in 24-36 hours
Type IV *(ID injection or Patch test)* an indurated red area, sometimes with vesiculation, developing within 24–48 hours and resolving over several days

Further reading
Pepys, J. (1975) *British Journal of Hospital Medicine,* **14,** 412.

Genetics

GLOSSARY OF TERMS

Alleles. Alternative forms of a gene occupying the same locus on homologous chromosomes. A child should receive one of each pair of alleles from each parent

Aneuploid. A chromosome number which is not an exact multiple of the haploid number

Autosome. Any chromosome other than the sex chromosomes. Man has 22 pairs of autosomes

Barr body. The sex chromatin seen in somatic cells of the female

Carrier. An individual who is heterozygous for a normal gene and an abnormal gene which is not expressed phenotypically

Chimera. An individual composed of cells from different zygotes. In 'blood-group' chimerism dyzygotic twins exchange haemopoietic stem cells in utero and continue to form blood cells of both types. In 'whole-body' chimerism two separate zygotes are fused into one individual

Chromatid. A chromosome consists of two parallel strands (chromatids) held together by the centromere

Clone. A cell line derived by mitosis from a single ancestral diploid cell

Concordant. A term used to describe a pair of twins in which both members exhibit a certain trait

Crossover. Exchange of genetic material between members of a chromosome pair

Deletion. A chromosomal aberration in which part of a chromosome is lost

Diploid. The number of chromosomes in somatic cells (which is double that of the gametes). In man this is 46

Discordant. A term used to describe a pair of twins in which one shows a certain trait and the other does not

Dizygotic. Twins produced by two ova, separately fertilised

Duplication. a chromosomal aberration in which part of a chromosome is duplicated

F1. The first generation progeny of a mating

Gametes. Reproductive cells which unite in pairs to form a zygote

Gene. A segment of DNA coded for the synthesis of a single polypeptide

Genome. (Genotype) The full set of genes

Haploid. the chromosome number of a normal gamete. In man this is 23

Hemizygous. A term applied to genes on the X chromosome in a male

Heterogeneity. A phenotype is genetically heterogeneous if it can be produced by different genetic mechanisms

Heterozygote. An individual with 2 different alleles at a given locus on a pair of homologous chromosomes

Holandric. The inheritance pattern of genes on a Y chromosome (i.e. transmitted to all sons but no daughters)

Homologous chromosomes. A 'matched pair' of chromosomes, one from each parent, having the same gene loci in the same order

Homozygote. An individual with 2 identical alleles at a given locus on a pair of homologous chromosomes

Inversion. A chromosomal aberration in which a segment of chromosome is inverted end-to-end

Isoalleles. 'Normal' alleles which can be distinguished from each other only by their differing phenotypic expression when in combination with a dominant mutant allele

Isochromosome. An abnormal chromosome with 2 arms of equal length, bearing the same loci in reverse sequence, formed by transverse (instead of longitudinal) division of the centromere

Karyotype. The chromosome set

Locus. The position of a gene on a chromosome

Mosaic. An individual or tissue with at least 2 cell lines differing in genotype

Multiple alleles. More than 2 alleles may occur at a given locus in a population even though each normal individual can have only 2 alleles at that locus

Penetrance. The frequency of expression of a genotype. A non-penetrant trait is not expressed in the phenotype

Phenotype. The individual produced by the interaction between the genotype and the environment

Pleiotropy. The production of multiple effects by a single gene

Polygenic. Determined by many genes at different loci, with small additive effects

Proband. (Propositus, index case.) The family member who first presents with a given trait

Recombination. The formation of new combinations of linked genes by crossing over between their loci

RNA. Ribonucleic acid, has 3 forms:

   (i) messenger RNA is the template for polypeptide synthesis
  (ii) transfer RNA brings activated amino-acids into position along this template
 (iii) ribosomal RNA is a component of ribosomes which functions as a non-specific site of polypeptide synthesis

Segregation. The separation of allelic genes at meiosis

Sex Chromatin. (Barr body) A chromatin mass in the nucleus which represents an inactive X chromosome. It is absent in the male

Sex-limited. A trait expressed only in one sex though the gene determining it is not X-linked

Sex-linked. A trait expressed by a gene on the X chromosome

Synteny. The presence of 2 or more gene loci on the same chromosome

Triplet. 3 successive bases in DNA or RNA which code for a specific amino-acid

Triploid. A cell or individual with 3 times the normal haploid chromosome number

Trisomy. The presence of 3 of a given chromosome instead of the usual pair, as in trisomy 21 (Down's)

Zygote. The fertilised ovum

Further reading

Thompson, J. & Thompson, M. (1973) *Genetics in Medicine,* p. 357. Philadelphia: Saunders.

HISTOCOMPATIBILITY (HL-A) ANTIGENS

Histocompatibility antigens are present on all tissues of the body. There are two series of antigens determined serologically at each of 2 loci, and a further series of antigens determined only in the mixed lymphocyte reaction. Some diseases occur more frequently in association with certain HL-A antigens, possibly due to related immune response (IR) genes.

The strongest association is between ankylosing spondylitis and B27

The following 'immunological' diseases are associated with B8:
1. Active chronic hepatitis
2. SLE
3. Sjøgren's disease
4. Juvenile dermatomyositis
5. Dermatitis herpetiformis
6. Coeliac disease
7. Graves' disease
8. Myasthenia gravis
9. Juvenile, insulin-dependent, diabetes mellitus
10. Addison's hypoadrenalism

Further reading

Sasazuki, T. et al (1977) *Annual Review of Medicine,* **28,** 425.
Voak, D. & Goldstone, A.H. (1976) *Hospital Update,* **2,** 483.

Microbiology

Causes of PUO
1. Infection
   (i) Exclude:
      tonsillitis, pneumonia, pyelonephritis, cholangitis, enteric fever, septicaemia, pus under tension, endocarditis, pericarditis, etc.
   (ii) Consider possibility of:
      TB, brucellosis, parasites (worms, malaria, etc.) and viral infections
2. Collagen-vascular disease
3. Malignancy (e.g. hypernephroma or lymphoma)
4. 'Silent' myocardial or pulmonary infarction
5. Drug hypersensitivity prior to onset of rash
6. Familial Mediterranean fever
7. Psychogenic and hysteria
8. Munchausen's syndrome

Gram staining of some important pathogens

Gram +ve	*Gram −ve*
Actinomyces	Brucella
Anthrax	Cholera
Clostridia	E. coli–Salmonella–Shigella
Coryn. diphtheriae	Haemophilus influenzae
Pneumococcus	Haemophilus pertussis
Staphylococcus	Klebsiella
Streptococcus	Neisseria (gonococcus, meningococc
TB	Pasteurella
	Pseudomonas
	Proteus
	Rickettsiae

Bactericidal drugs	**Bacteriostatic drugs**
Penicillins, cephalosporins	Sulphonamides
Streptomycin, neomycin	Tetracyclines
Kanamycin	Chloramphenicol
Co-trimoxazole	Erythromycin
Polymyxin, colistin	Novobiocin
Isoniazid	PAS
Bacitracin	Lincomycin, clindamycin
Metronidazole	
Aminoglycosides (tobramycin and gentamycin)	

Organisms virtually always sensitive to penicillin
Strep. pyogenes (Gp.A)
Strep. pneumoniae (pneumococcus)
Neisseria meningitidis
Treponema pallidum

CLASSIFICATION OF SOME COMMON VIRUSES
RNA containing viruses
 1. *Picornaviruses*
        (i) Enteroviruses
              Polio
              Echo
              Coxsackie
       (ii) Rhinoviruses
              Coryza etc.
 2. *Myxoviruses and paramyxoviruses*
            Influenza
            Mumps
            Measles
            Respiratory syncytial
 3. *Reoviruses*
            Upper respiratory tract infections
 4. *Arborviruses*
            Endemic encephalitis
            Yellow fever
            Dengue
            Sandfly fever
 5. *Rhabdoviruses*
            Rabies

DNA containing viruses
 1. *Poxviruses*
            Variola
            Vaccinia
            Molluscum contagiosum
            Orf
 2. *Adenoviruses*
            Upper respiratory tract infections
            Conjunctivitis, etc.
 3. *Herpesviruses*
            Herpesvirus hominis (H. simplex)
            Varicella-zoster
            Epstein Barr virus
            Cytomegalic inclusion disease
 4. *Papillomaviruses*
            Verruca vulgaris

Clinical chemistry

NORMAL ADULT RANGE FOR LABORATORY ASSAYS

The International System of Units (SI units) has now been widely introduced in British laboratories in place of the traditional Imperial Units, which were empirical. SI units are preferred by the Royal Colleges for examination questions, but at present Imperial Units are also given in parentheses. It is likely that eventually SI Units only will be quoted. Submultiples of SI units use the following prefixes:

Factor	Name	Symbol
10^{-1}	deci	d
10^{-2}	centi	c
10^{-3}	milli	m
10^{-6}	micro	μ
10^{-9}	nano	n
10^{-12}	pico	p
10^{-15}	femto	f

Even with SI units, values may vary in different laboratories.

Further reading

Paterson, N. & Fraser, S.C. (1975) *British Journal of Hospital Medicine,* **13,** 757.

Blood

Acid phosphatase, 1–3.5 KA units/100 ml
    (Tartrate labile, up to 0.8 KA units/100 ml)
Alanine amino-transferase, up to 45 Reitman-Frankel units/ml
Alkaline phosphatase, 25–85 IU/100 ml (3–13 KA units/100 ml)
Ammonium, 23–47 μmol/l (40–80 μg/100 ml)
Amylase, up to 200 Somogyi units
Ascorbic acid, 34–114 μmol/l (0.6–2.0 mg/100 ml)
Aspartate amino-transferase, up to 50 Reitman-Frankel units/ml
B_{12}, 100–1000 ng/l(or $\mu\mu$g/ml)
Bilirubin (total), up to 17 μmol/l (up to 1 mg/100 ml)
Calcium, 2.2–2.7 mmol/l (9.0–10.8 mg/100 ml)
    Ionized calcium, 1.1–2.4 mmol/l (4.5–5.6 mg/100 ml)
Cholesterol, 3.6–6.7 mmol/l (140–260 mg/100 ml)
Cholinesterase, 2–4 units
Copper, 12–25 μmol/l (75–160 μg/100 ml)
Copper oxidase, 0.20–0.55 units
Cortisol, (11-hydroxycorticosteroids)
    9 am, 190–690 nmol/l (7–25 μg/100 ml)
    12 midnight, 80–190 nmol/l (3–7 μg/100 ml)

Creatinine, 53–106 μmol/l (0.6–1.2 mg/100 ml)
Electrolytes
    Na, 136–149 mmol/l (or mEq/l)
    K, 3.8–5.2 mmol/l (or mEq/l)
    Cl, 100–107 mmol/l (or mEq/l)
    Bicarb, 24–30 mmol/l (or mEq/l)
Fibrinogen, 2–4 g/l (200–400 mg/100 ml)
Folate, 6–21 μg/l (or mμg/ml)
Glucose (fasting venous sample, glucose oxidase assay),
    3.0–5.3 mmol/l (55–95 mg/100 ml)
Haptoglobin, 0.7–1.3 g/l (72–125 mg/100 ml)
HGH, 1–5 μlU/ml during G.T.T.
Immunoglobulins
    IgG, 80–160 mg/l
    IgA, 14–42 mg/l
    IgM, 5–19 mg/l
    IgD, 0.03–4 mg/l
Iron
    Males, 14–32 μmol/l (80–180 μg/100 ml)
    Females, 11–29 μmol/l (60–160 μg/100 ml)
Lactic dehydrogenase, 55–200 IU/l (110–400
    spectrophotometric units/ml)
5-Nucleotidase, 1.6–17.0 IU/l
Phosphate, 0.8–1.4 mmol/l (2.5–4.5 mg/100 ml)
Protein (total), 60–80 g/l (6–8 g/100 ml)
    Albumin, 33–46 g/l (3.3–4.6 g/100 ml)
    α1 globulin, 1–4 g/l (0.1–0.4 g/100 ml)
    α2 globulin, 5–10 g/l (0.5–1.0 g/100 ml)
    β globulin, 6–11 g/l (0.6–1.1 g/100 ml)
    γ globulin; 6–12 g/l (0.6–1.2 g/100 ml)
Protein-bound iodine, 236–550 nmol/l (3.0–7.0 μg/100 ml)
Red cell folate, 160–640 μg/l (or mμg/ml)
Thymol turbidity, 0–4 units
Thyroxine 70–160 nmol/l
TIBC, 45– 72 μmol/l (250–400 μg/100 ml)
Triglycerides (fasting) 0.3–1.7 mmol/l
Urea, 2.5–6.6 mmol/l (15–40 mg/100 ml)
Uric acid, up to 0.4 mmol/l (up to 6 mg/100 ml)

Blood gases (arterial)
Oxygen 12–15 k Pa (90–100 mmHg)
Carbon dioxide 4.5–6.1 k Pa (34–46 mmHg)

Urine (assuming a normal diet)
Specific gravity 1.008–1.030
pH 4.8–7.5
Ascorbic acid, 114–170 μmol/24 h (20–30 mg/24 hr)
Calcium, 2.5–7.5 mmol/24 (100–300 mg/24 hr)
Chloride, 100–180 mmol/24 h (or mEq/24 hr)
Creatinine, 9–17 mmol/24 h (1–2 g/24 hr)
5HIAA, 16–73 μmol/24 h (3–14 mg/24 hr)
Phosphate, 16–48 mmol/24 h (0.5–1.5 g/24 hr)
Potassium, 25–100 mmol/24 h (or mEq/24 hr)
Sodium, 100–200 mmol/24 h (or mEq/24 hr)
VMA, 10–40 μmol/24 h (2–8 mg/24 hr)
17-Hydroxycorticoids (Porter-Silber),
    Male 3–10 mg/24 hr
    Female 2–6 mg/24 hr
17-Ketosteroids,
    Male 9–22 mg/24 hr
    Female 6–15 mg/24 hr
Urea 250–500 mmol/l (10–40 g/24 hr)

CSF
Chloride, 120–128 mmol/l (or mEq/l)
Glucose, 2.5–3.9 mmol/l (45–70 mg/100 ml)
Protein, up to 0.4 g/l (up to 40 mg/100 ml)
Lymphocytes, up to 4/cu mm

SPECIAL TESTS
Glucose tolerance test
Normal limits, using 50 g oral load with capillary samples and
reduction method of assay
  1. Fasting true blood glucose does not exceed 6.7 mmol/l (120
     mg/100 ml)
  2. Blood glucose does not rise above 8.9 mmol/l (160 mg/100 ml)
  3. Blood glucose returns below 6.7 mmol/l (120 mg/100 ml
     within 2 hr)

'Maximal' gastric secretion test
Using pentagastrin 6μg/kg IM

Basal sample (60 min)	*Post-pentagastrin samples (60 min)*
Females: 1–2 mEq/hr	10–20 mEq/hr
Males: 2–3 mEq/hr	15–25 mEq/hr

Creatinine clearance should exceed 100 ml/min

Ammonium chloride test for urinary acidification
(using 0.1 g/kg body wt of NH_4Cl)
Urine pH should fall below 5.3 and urinary titratable acidity should
exceed 25 μEq/min

Phosphate excretion index (PEI)

The ratio $\dfrac{\text{phosphate clearance}}{\text{creatinine clearance}}$ is dependent upon the plasma PO_4 level.

The PEI indicates the extent to which this ratio departs from the predicted normal for a given plasma PO_4 level.

i.e. $PEI = \text{Observed } \dfrac{CP}{CCr} - \text{'Normal' } \dfrac{CP}{CCr}$

where the normal $\dfrac{CP}{CCr} = 0.055 \text{ plasma } PO_4 - 0.07$.

On a normal diet, PEI should be 0 ± 0.09

BSP excretion test (using 5 mg/kg)
Not more than 5 per cent BSP should remain in the blood at 45 minutes
Xylose absorption test (using 25 g xylose)
The 5 hour urinary excretion of xylose should exceed 6 g
Fat absorption test on normal diet
Total faecal fat over 5 days should not exceed 5 g/day

Dexamethasone suppression test

1. Dexamethasone 0.5 mg 6 hourly for 2 days
   Normally urinary 17-Hydroxycorticoids suppress to less than 2.5 mg/24 hr
   In adrenocortical hyperplasia there is less suppression
2. Dexamethasone 2.0 mg 6 hourly for 2 days
   With bilateral hyperplasia there is suppression to less than 50% of the base-line assay
   With adenoma or carcinoma there is less suppression

Note that exceptions may occur

Synacthen test

Plasma cortisol (11-OHCS) is measured before and 30 min after 250 µg Synacthen IM
   The initial cortisol conc should exceed 138 nmol/l (5 µg/100 ml)
At 30 min the cortisol conc should exceed 495 nmol/l (18 µg/100 ml) and the increment (irrespective of the initial level) should exceed 193 nmol/l (7 µg/100 ml)

Insulin tolerance tests (Dangerous in hypopituitarism)

Standard. After an overnight fast, soluble insulin is given IV in a dose of 0.1 U/kg and blood glucose, cortisol and GH are measured every 30 min for 2 hr. GH conc should exceed 10 µlU/ml in at least one post-insulin specimen.
Augmented ITT (for acromegaly) uses 0.3 U/kg and should not be performed if hypopituitarism is suspected

Bibliography

It is unlikely that even the most assiduous of candidates will find time to study all of the following books. Special attention should be paid to the subjects in which the least clinical experience has been gained.
Asterisks denote larger texts and reference books

Cardiology
Schamroth, L. (1971) *An Introduction to Electrocardiography,* 4th edn. Oxford: Blackwell.
Schire, V. (1977) *Clinical Cardiology,* 3rd. edn. London: Granada
*Goldman, M.J. (1976) *Principles of Clinical Electrocardiography* 9th edn. Los Altos: Lange.
*Hurst, J.W. (1974) *The Heart, Arteries and Veins,* 3rd edn. Kogakusha, Tokyo: McGraw-Hill.

Chest disease
Cole, R.B. (1975) *Essentials of Respiratory Disease,* 2nd edn. London: Pitman.
*Crofton, J. & Douglas, A. (1975) *Respiratory Diseases,* 2nd edn. Oxford: Blackwell.

Gastro-enterology
Naish, J.M. & Read, A.E. (1974) *Basic Gastroenterology,* 2nd edn. Bristol: Wright.
*Sherlock, Sheila. (1975) *Diseases of the Liver and Biliary System,* 5th edn. Oxford: Blackwell.
*Sleisenger, M.H. & Fordtran, J.S. (1973) *Gastro-intestinal Disease.* Philadelphia: W.B. Saunders.

Haematology
*Hardisty, R.M. & Weatherall, D.J. (1974) *Blood and its Disorders.* Oxford: Blackwell.
Hoffbrand, A.V. & Lewis, S.M. (1972) *Haematology. Tutorials in Postgraduate Medicine,* Vol. 2. London: Heinemann.

Neurology
*Merrit, H.H. (1973) *A Textbook of Neurology,* 5th edn. Philadelphia: Lea & Febiger.
Walton, J.N. (1975) *Essentials of Neurology,* 4th edn. London: Pitman.

Endocrine and bone disease
Hall, R., Anderson, J., Smart, G.A. & Besser, M. (1974) *Fundamentals of Clinical Endocrinology,* 2nd edn. London: Pitman.

*Nordin, B.E.C. (1973) *Metabolic Bone and Stone Disease.*
    Edinburgh: Churchill Livingstone.
*Williams, R.H. (1974) *Textbook of Endocrinology,* 5th edn.
    Philadelphia: Saunders.

Renal disease
Gabriel, R. (1977) *Postgraduate Nephrology.* 2nd. edn. London:
    Butterworth.
*Strauss, M.B. & Welt, L.H. (1972) *Diseases of the Kidney,* 2nd edn.
    Edinburgh: Churchill Livingstone.

Rheumatology
Hughes, G.R.V. (1977) *Connective Tissue Diseases.* Oxford:
    Blackwell.
*Katz, W.A. (1977) *Rheumatic Diseases, Diagnosis and
    Management.* Philadelphia: Lippincott.

Immunology
Taylor, G. (1975) *Immunology in Clinical Practice.* London:
    Saunders.

Dermatology
Marks, R. & Samman, P.D. (1977) *Dermatology. Tutorials in
    Postgraduate Medicine,* Vol. 6. London: Heineman
*Rook, A., Wilkinson, D.S. & Ebling, F.J.G. (1972) *Textbook of
    Dermatology,* 2nd edn. Oxford: Blackwell.

Venereology
King, A. & Nicol, C. (1975) *Venereal Diseases,* 3rd edn. London:
    Baillière Tindall.

Clinical chemistry
Zilva, J.F. & Pannall, P.R. (1975) *Clinical Chemistry in Diagnosis and
    Treatment,* 2nd edn. London: Lloyd-Luke.

Common acute poisoning
Matthew, H. & Lawson, A.A.H. (1975) *Treatment of Common Acute
    Poisonings,* 3rd edn. Edinburgh: Churchill Livingstone.

Psychiatry
*Mayer-Gross, W., Slater, E. & Roth, M. (1969) *Clinical Psychiatry,*
    3rd edn. London: Baillière, Tindall & Cassell.

Rodger, T.F., Ingram, I.M., Timbury, G.C. & Mowbray, R.M. (1972)
    Lecture Notes on Psychiatric Medicine, 3rd edn. Edinburgh:
    Churchill Livingstone.

Paediatrics
Brimblecombe, F. & Barltrop D. (1978) *Children in Health and
    Disease.* London: Ballière, Tindall & Cassell.

General

Bloom, A., Beck, E., Davies, P.D.B., Hoffbrand, B.I., Sharland, D.E. (1976) *Whittington Postgraduate Medicine.* London: Butterworth.

Bomford, R.R., Mason, S. & Swash, M. (1975) *Hutchison's Clinical Methods,* 16th edn. London: Baillière Tindall.

Burton, J.L. (1976) *Aids to Undergraduate Medicine,* 2nd edn. Edinburgh: Churchill Livingstone.

Davies, I.J.T. (1977) *Postgraduate Medicine,* 3rd edn. London: Lloyd-Luke.

Macleod, J. (1976) *Clinical Examination,* 4th edn. Edinburgh: Churchill Livingstone.

Spalton, D.J., Sever, P.S. & Ward, P.D. (1976) *100 Case Histories for the M.R.C.P.* Edinburgh: Churchill Livingstone.

*Beeson, P.D. & McDermott, W. (1975) *Cecil Loeb Textbook of Medicine,* 14th edn. Philadelphia: Saunders.

*Hunter, D. (1975) *The Diseases of Occupations,* 5th edn. London: English Universities Press.

Journals
Excellent review articles suitable for M.R.C.P. candidates appear regularly in Medicine, Hospital Update and the British Journal of Hospital Medicine. Relevant leading articles in the British Medical Journal, The Lancet and the New England Journal of Medicine should also be read. These latter journals also contain many important original papers, and though one cannot read every paper in detail it is worth scanning each issue to pick out advances relating to internal medicine. Every reader must develop a method which suits him best, but I find that the quickest way to imprint the 'message' of a paper on my memory is to read the Summary, then the Introduction (which puts the work in perspective and explains why it was done), and then re-read the Summary. Examination candidates are unlikely to have time to read the Methodology and Discussion of original papers except in subjects in which they have a special interest. In any case it is unwise to be too critical of a paper in the M.R.C.P. examination as you may be speaking to its author.

Index

Abdominal pain, 58
Absent jerks with extensor plantars, 112
Absent spleen, 81
Acid-base balance, 149
Acidosis, 149, 150
Active chronic hepatitis, 49
A.D.H., 152
Adrenal hyperplasia, 122
Adrenal insufficiency, 122
Alcohol, 93
Aldosterone, 123
Alkalosis, 149
Allergic reactions, 183
Alpha-fetoprotein, 51
Amenorrhoea, 126
Amino-aciduria, 147
Ammonium chloride test, 196
Anaemia 66-71
Angiotensin, 123
Ankylosing spondylitis, 162, 163
Anticoagulants, 90
Antinuclear antibodies, 157
Aplastic anaemia, 72
Arginine vasopressin, 152
Argyll Robertson pupils, 112
Arrhythmias, 10, 11
Arterial pulse, 10
Arteritis, 159
Atrial fibrillation, 11
Atrophic spleen, 81

Bactericidal drugs, 192
Bacteriostatic drugs, 192
Basal arteries of brain, 100
Behcet's syndrome, 182
Bibliography, 198 -200
Biochemical tests, 194 - 197
Biological false positive W.R., 166
Bleeding, 85 - 88
Blindness, 92, 105
Blood gases, 22, 195
Blood transfusion, 91
B lymphocytes, 184, 185
Bone disease, 133, 136
Bone metastases, 35
Bradycardia, 10
Bronchial carcinoma, 33
Bronchitis, 25
Broncho-pulmonary segments, 20

Brudzinski's test, 117
BSP excretion, 197
Bulbar palsy, 94
Bundle branch block, 19

Calcification, abdominal, 57
Calcification, soft tissue, 136
Calcium pyrophosphate arthropathy, 162, 164
Carcino-embryonic antigen, 62
Carcinoma bronchus, 33
Carcinoma, non-metastatic complications, 33, 110, 167
Carcinomatous neuropathy, 110
Cardiac axis, 17
Cardiomegaly, 14
Cardiomyopathy, 13
Carpal tunnel syndrome, 161
Cataract, 103
Cerebro-spinal fluid, 196
Cervical sympathetic pathway, 104
Charcot joint, 112
Chondrocalcinosis, 162, 164
Cigarette smoking, 26
Cirrhosis, 46
Clubbing, 34
Coagulation, 86 - 89
Coma, 97
Complement, 187
Compliance, 23
Congenital adrenal hyperplasia, 122
Connective tissue disorders, 165
Constipation, 40
Cord compression, 107
Cor pulmonale, 27
Crackles, 24
Crohn's disease, 60
Cryoglobulinaemia, 154

Dark urine, 147
Dementia, 96
Dermatomes, 110
Dexamethasone suppression test, 197
Diabetes mellitus
  and pregnancy, 120
  causes, 118
  complications, 119
  definition, 118
Dialysis, 139

Diaphragm, 106
Diarrhoea, 41
Diffusion, 22
Disseminated CNS lesions, 95
Disseminated intravascular
    coagulation, 89
Dropped beats, 10
Drug-induced haemolysis, 68
Drug-induced liver disease, 53
Drug-induced pulmonary disease, 29
Drug-induced renal disease, 148
Drug-induced skin disease, 178
Drug interactions, 54
Dysarthria, 94
Dysphagia, 36

Electrocardiography, 17
Emphysema, 25
Encephalopathy, hepatic, 48
Eosinophilia, 74
Epilepsy, 95
Excretion urography, 145
Eye movements, 104

Facial nerve, 98
Facial pain, 98
Familial jaundice, 55
Fanconi syndrome, 146
Fibrinogen deficiency, 89
Folate deficiency, 69
Frontal 'bossing', 136

Galactorrhoea, 125
Gastrectomy complications, 56
Gastric secretion, 55, 196
Genetic terms, 188
Giddiness, 99
Gingival swelling, 38
G6P dehydrogenase def., 69
Glomerulonephritis, 140
Glucose tolerance test, 118, 196
Glycogen storage disease, 116
Gonorrhoea, 181
Gout, 162, 163
Gram stains, 192
Gut flora, 44
Gut hormones, 62
Gynaecomastia, 125

Haematemesis, 56
Haemochromatosis, 52
Haemodialysis, 139
Haemolytic anaemia, 67
Haemophilia, 87
Haemosiderosis, 52
Headache, 97

Heart,
    block, 11
    failure, 7
    murmurs, 4
    sounds, 3
Heinz bodies, 65
Hemianopia, 101
Hepatitis, 49
Hepatolenticular degeneration, 52
Hepatomegaly, 44
Hirsutism, 176
HLA antigens, 191
Hodgkin's disease, 75
Howell-Jolly bodies, 65
Hypercalcaemia
    causes, 134
    ECG changes, 19
Hypercalciuria, 135
Hyperdynamic circulation, 16
Hypergammaglobulinaemia, 185
Hyperkalaemia
    ECG changes, 19
Hyperlipoproteinaemia, 171
Hypermobile joints, 160
Hypernatraemia, 151
Hyperparathyroidism, 135
Hypersplenism, 81
Hypertension
    portal, 47
    pulmonary, 12
    systemic, 12, 123
Hyperthyroidism, 129
Hypertrichosis, 177
Hypertrophic osteoarthropathy, 34
Hyperuricaemia, 163
Hyperventilation, 23
Hypoadrenalism, 122
Hypocalcaemia
    causes, 134
    ECG causes, 19
Hypochlorhydria, 55
Hypochromic anaemia, 66
Hypogammaglobulinaemia, 185
Hypoglycaemia, 121
Hypokalaemia, 19, 150
Hypomelanosis, 175
Hyponatraemia, 151
Hypoparathyroidism, 134
Hypoprothrombinaemia, 90
Hypothalamic hormones, 132
Hypothyroidism, 129
Hypoventilation, 23

Immunoglobulins, 185
Immune deficiency, 185-187
Inclusion bodies, 65

Industrial chest disease, 27
Industrial skin disease, 180
Innocent murmurs, 6
Insulin tolerance test, 197
Intersexual states, 128
Interstitial nephritis, 142
Intestinal polyps, 61
Irregular pulse, 10, 11

Jaundice
    drug induced, 53
    familial non-haemolytic, 55
    with uraemia, 151
JVP, 9

Kernig's test, 117
Kidneys, large, 145
Kidneys, small, 145

Lactic acidosis, 150
Laryngeal nerves, 106
Lead poisoning, 66
Leucocytosis, 73
Leuco-erythroblastic anaemia, 73
Leucopenia, 72
Leukaemias, 77
Leukaemoid reaction, 73
Lipoproteins, 171
Liver tumours, 50
Lung abscess, 30
Lung anatomy, 20
Lung volumes, 21
Lupus erythematosus, 157
Lymphocytosis, 74
Lymphomas, 76

Machinery murmur, 5
Macrocytic anaemia, 69-71
Malabsorption, 42
Malignancy,
    complications, 33
    metastases, 35
    skin changes, 167
Marrow depression, 71
Mass in R iliac fossa, 57
Mediastinal masses, 36
Megaloblastic anaemia, 69
Metabolic bone disease, 133
Metastases, 35
Microangiopathic haemolytic
        anaemia, 68
Monocytosis, 74
Mononeuritis multiplex, 109
MRCP examination, 1
Mucopolysaccharides, 165

Multiple endocrine adenomatosis,
        137
Murmurs, 4-6
Muscular dystrophy, 116
Myeloproliferative disease, 78
Myocardial infarction,
    complications, 14
    ECG changes, 18
Myopathy, 115
Myotonia, 114

Nails, 177
Nephrocalcinosis, 143, 144
Nephrotic syndrome, 141
Neurological complications of:
    carcinoma, 110
    diabetes mellitus, 119
    renal failure, 139
Neurological terms, 92
Neuromuscular transmission, 114
Neurosyphilis, 112
Neutropenia, 72
Non-Hodgkin's lymphoma, 76
'Normal' chest X-ray, 30
Normal values,
    biochemical, 194-197
    haematological, 63
Nuclear fluorescence, 158
Nystagmus, 99

Opening snap, 3
Optic atrophy, 102
Optic neuritis, 102
Osteoarthrosis, 162
Osteomalacia, 133
Osteoporosis, 133
Ovarian tumours, 127

Palmar erythema, 179
Pancreatitis, 57
Pancytopenia, 72
Papillary necrosis, 142
Papillitis, 104
Papilloedema, 104
Pappenheimer bodies, 65
Paraplegia, 107
Parenteral nutrition, 61
Parkinsonism, 113
Parotid enlargement, 40
Peptic ulcer, 56
Percussion, 24
Pericarditis, 16
Periosteal reaction, 162
Peripheral nerves, 108, 109
Phaeochromocytoma, 137
Phagocyte deficiency, 186

Phosphate excretion index, 135, 197
Photosensitivity, 173
Pigmentation, 174
Platelet defect: , 82-84
Pleural effusion, 31
Pneumoconiosis, 29
Pneumonia, slow resolution, 27
Pneumothorax, 31
Polycythaemia, 79, 139
Polydipsia, 152
Polyps, intestinal, 61
Polyuria, 152
Porphyria, 169, 170
Porta-caval shunt, 47
Portal hypertension, 47
Post. inf. cerebellar thrombosis, 100
Precocious puberty, 128
Prostaglandins, 126
Protein-losing enteropathy, 58
Pruritis, 179
Pseudo-bulbar palsy, 94
Pseudogout, 162, 164
Ptosis, 104
Pulmonary,
    commonly confused signs, 24
    compliance, 23
    diffusion, 22
    fibrosis, 28
    hypertension, 12
    metastases, 35
    oedema, 32
Pulse, 10, 11
Pyrexia of unknown origin, 192
Pyuria, 142

Radiology,
    chest, 14, 28, 30
    joints, 162
    kidneys, 145
    skull, 136
Ramsay-Hunt syndrome, 98
Raynaud's phenomenon, 153
Recurrent laryngeal nerves, 106
Red cell inclusion bodies, 65
Red cell shape, 64
Reiter's syndrome, 182
Renal calculi, 143
Renal failure, 138
Renal tubular disorders, 146
Renal veinthrombosis, 141
Renin, 123
Retinal haemorrhage, 105
Retrobulbar neuritis, 102
Rheumatoid disease, 154-156, 162
Rheumatoid factor, 156
Rickets, 133

Rye classification, 75

Sarcoidosis, 35
Scotoma, 101
Scleroderma, 168
Secondary syphilis, 181
Shoulder-hand syndrome, 161
Sideroblastic anaemia, 66
SI units, 194
Sjogren's syndrome, 156
Skin changes in malignancy, 167
Skin tests, 187
SLE criteria, 157
Soft-tissue calcification, 136
Spirometry, 21
Splenectomy, 81
Splenomegaly, 80
Spinal cord, 106
Steroid side-effects, 124
Stevens-Johnson syndrome, 182
Stiffness, 160
Stomatitis, 38
Stones, renal, 143
Straight-leg raising, 117
Superficial reflexes, 106
Synacthen test, 197
Syncope, 15
Syphilis, 112, 181

Tachycardia, 10
TBG, 131
Tendon reflexes, 106
Textbooks, 198-200
Thalassaemia, 69
Thomas' test, 117
Thoracic outlet syndromes, 161
Thrombocytopenia, 82
Thrombocytosis, 84
Thrombosis, 84
Thyroid function tests, 130, 131
Tibial 'bowing', 136
T lymphocytes, 184, 186
Transfusion, 91
Transient ischaemic attacks, 105
Translucencies in skull X-ray, 136
Tremor, 113
Triple rhythm, 3
Tunnel vision, 101
T waves, 18

Ulcerative colitis, 59
Uveitis, 103

Vagotomy, 56
Valsalva manoeuvre, 7
Valvular disease, 7

Vasculitis, 159
Venous pulse, 9
Ventricular failure, 8
Ventricular hypertrophy, 17
Vertigo, 99
Vessel defects, 85
Virus classification, 193
Visual defects, 101
Vital capacity, 21
Vitamin deficiency
    B_{12}, 70
    D, 133
    K, 90

Vitiligo, 175
Vocal resonance, 24
Vomiting, 39
von Willebrand's disease, 87

Wasting of hand muscles, 108
Wheezes, 23
WR, 166

Xanthomas, 171